Physical Therapy Management of Parkinson's Disease

CLINICS IN PHYSICAL THERAPY

EDITORIAL BOARD

Otto D. Payton, Ph.D., **Chairman**
Louis R. Amundsen, Ph.D.
Suzann K. Campbell, Ph.D.

Already Published

Rehabilitation of the Burn Patient
Vincent R. DiGregorio, M.D., guest editor

Spinal Cord Injury
Hazel V. Adkins, M.A., R.P.T., guest editor

Measurement in Physical Therapy
Jules M. Rothstein, Ph.D., guest editor

Hand Rehabilitation
Christine A. Moran, M.S., R.P.T., guest editor

Sports Physical Therapy
Donna Bernhardt, M.S., R.P.T., A.T.C., guest editor

Pain
John L. Echternach, Ed.D., guest editor

Physical Therapy of the Low Back
Lance T. Twomey, Ph.D., and James R. Taylor, M.D.,
Ph.D., guest editors

Therapeutic Considerations for the Elderly
Osa Littrup Jackson, Ph.D., guest editor

Physical Therapy of the Foot and Ankle
Gary C. Hunt, M.A., P.T., guest editor

Physical Therapy Management of Arthritis
Barbara Banwell, M.A., P.T., and Victoria Gall, M.Ed.,
P.T., guest editors

**Physical Therapy of the Cervical and
Thoracic Spine**
Ruth Grant, M.App.Sc., Grad.Dip.Adv.Man.Ther.,
guest editor

**TMJ Disorders: Management of the
Craniomandibular Complex**
Steven L. Kraus, P.T., guest editor

Physical Therapy of the Knee
Robert E. Mangine, M.Ed., P.T., A.T.C., guest editor

**Obstetric and Gynecologic Physical
Therapy**
Elaine Wilder, R.P.T., M.A.C.T., guest editor

**Physical Therapy of the Geriatric Patient,
2nd Ed.**
Osa L. Jackson, Ph.D., R.P.T., guest editor

Physical Therapy for the Cancer Patient
Charles L. McGarvey III, M.S., P.T., guest editor

Gait in Rehabilitation
Gary L. Smidt, Ph.D., guest editor

Physical Therapy of the Hip
John L. Echternach, Ed.D., guest editor

Physical Therapy of the Shoulder, 2nd Ed.
Robert Donatelli, M.A., P.T., guest editor

Pediatric Neurologic Physical Therapy, 2nd Ed.
Suzann K. Campbell, Ph.D., P.T., F.A.P.T.A., guest editor

Forthcoming Volumes in the Series

**Pulmonary Management in Physical
Therapy**
Cynthia C. Zadai, M.S., P.T., guest editor

Physical Therapy Assessment in Early Infancy
Irma J. Wilhelm, M.S., P.T., guest editor

Physical Therapy of the Low Back, 2nd Ed.
Lance T. Twomey, Ph.D., and James R. Taylor, M.D., Ph. D., guest editors

Physical Therapy Management of Parkinson's Disease

Edited by
George I. Turnbull, M.A., P.T.

Associate Professor and Chair
Department of Physical Therapy
University of South Alabama College of Allied Health Professions
Mobile, Alabama
Associate Professor
Dalhousie University School of Physiotherapy
Halifax, Nova Scotia, Canada

CHURCHILL LIVINGSTONE
New York, Edinburgh, London, Melbourne, Tokyo

Library of Congress Cataloging-in-Publication Data
Physical therapy management of Parkinson's disease / edited by George
  I. Turnbull.
        p.   cm. — (Clinics in physical therapy)
     Includes bibliographical references and index.
     ISBN 0-443-08756-3
     1. Parkinsonism—Physical therapy. I. Turnbull, George I.
  II.   Series.
     [DNLM: 1. Parkinson Disease—rehabilitation. 2. Physical Therapy.
  WL 359 P578]
  RC382.P59 1992
  616.8'33062—dc20
  DNLM/DLC
  for Library of Congress   92-13649
                                                               CIP

© **Churchill Livingstone Inc. 1992**

Distributed in the United Kingdom by Churchill Livingstone, Robert Stevenson
House, 1–3 Baxter's Place, Leith Walk, Edinburgh EH1 3AF, and by associated companies, branches, and representatives throughout the world.

Accurate indications, adverse reactions, and dosage schedules for drugs are
provided in this book, but it is possible that they may change. The reader is
urged to review the package information data of the manufacturers of the medications mentioned.

The Publishers have made every effort to trace the copyright holders for bor-
rowed material. If they have inadvertently overlooked any, they will be pleased
to make the necessary arrangements at the first opportunity.

Acquisitions Editor: *Leslie Burgess*
Copy Editor: *Elizabeth Bowman-Schulman*
Production Designer: *Jody L. Ouellette*
Production Supervisor: *Jeanine Furino*

Printed in the United States of America

First published in 1992   7 6 5 4 3 2 1

Contributors

Susan E. Doble, M.S.
Assistant Professor, Dalhousie University School of Occupational Therapy, Halifax, Nova Scotia, Canada

Alan Fine, V.M.D., Ph.D.
Associate Professor, Department of Physiology and Biophysics, Dalhousie University Faculty of Medicine; Assistant Professor, Division of Neurology, Department of Medicine, Victoria General Hospital, Halifax, Nova Scotia, Canada

John D. Fisk, Ph.D.
Honourary Adjunct Assistant Professor, Department of Psychiatry, Dalhousie University Faculty of Medicine; Coordinator, Neuropsychology Services, Camp Hill Medical Centre, Halifax, Nova Scotia, Canada

Roy A. Fox, M.D.
Professor and Head, Division of Geriatric Medicine, Department of Medicine, Dalhousie University Faculty of Medicine; Director, Center for Health Care of the Elderly, Camp Hill Medical Centre, Halifax, Nova Scotia, Canada

David B. King, M.D.
Assistant Professor, Division of Neurology, Department of Medicine, Dalhousie University Faculty of Medicine; Director, Movement Disorder Clinic, Victoria General Hospital, Halifax, Nova Scotia, Canada

James G. Phillips
Reader, Psychology Department, Monash University, Clayton, Victoria, Australia

Douglas D. Rasmusson, Ph.D.
Professor, Department of Physiology and Biophysics, Dalhousie University Faculty of Medicine, Halifax, Nova Scotia, Canada

Margaret Schenkman, Ph.D., P.T.
Associate Professor, Graduate Program in Physical Therapy, and Senior Fellow, Center for the Study of Aging and Human Development, Duke University; Director, Posture and Balance Laboratory, Veterans Administration Medical Center, Durham, North Carolina

viii   *Contributors*

Margaret H. Sharpe, Ph.D., M. Sc., M.A.P.A.
Senior Lecturer, Department of Neurological Physiotherapy, University of South Australia School of Physiotherapy, Adelaide, South Australia, Australia

George E. Stelmach, Ph.D.
Professor, Departments of Exercise Science and Psychology, Arizona State University College of Liberal Arts and Sciences, Tempe, Arizona

George I. Turnbull, M.A., P.T.
Associate Professor and Chair, Department of Physical Therapy, University of South Alabama College of Allied Health Professions, Mobile, Alabama; Associate Professor, Dalhousie University School of Physiotherapy, Halifax, Nova Scotia, Canada

James C. Wall, Ph.D.
Professor, Department of Physical Therapy, University of South Alabama College of Allied Health Professions, Mobile, Alabama

Preface

Physical therapy is a profession in which expertise in problem-solving is of considerable importance. Attempts are made during the educational process to instill this critical competency, and most physical therapy educational programs try to recruit individuals who possess this trait. However, many of the books about physical therapy attempt to provide definitive answers to clinical problems. This occurs despite the fact that little in the field has been researched and even less is known, for certain, about the solutions to various problems.

Physical Therapy Management of Parkinson's Disease has been written from the standpoint that we do not know exactly how to manage Parkinson's disease (PD). Instead, the book asks questions, suggests answers, and presents a number of diverse perspectives. This has been done to encourage thought and constructive discussion and to facilitate the problem-solving skills of the practicing physical therapist so that rational clinical decisions relevant to the needs of a given patient can be constructed. Similarly, it is hoped that possible solutions to many of the issues raised will be generated and later researched in a manner appropriate for a responsible professional group. It is only through subscription to this mindset that viable solutions will be developed.

We hope that those physical therapists who read this book will use its content to attain a deeper understanding of the problems that face the PD patient and attempt to find successful answers. This will require problem-solving capabilities and creativity, both of which are major reasons why physical therapy is a dynamic and exciting profession.

The ultimate objective of this book is to better serve the PD population with methods developed by physical therapists for physical therapists. However, this must be done with the clear understanding that the physical therapist is but one of many players who can contribute to the well being of this clinical group. As the medical and surgical management of the disorder continue to progress, the physical therapy community must clearly establish the nature of a meaningful role as it has done in the care of other neurologic disorders, such as stroke. As the number of elderly in the population steadily increases and the prevalence of PD grows, we hope that this book will help attain that objective not by providing presumptuous answers but by providing the background to permit each and every physical therapist to exercise rational judgment, thereby achieving effective management of this difficult condition.

George I. Turnbull, M.A., P.T.

Acknowledgments

I wish to acknowledge the Nova Scotia Division of the Parkinson Foundation of Canada for substantially contributing to the motivation that eventually led to the production of this book. Particular thanks are due to Moira and Peter, who truly have been an inspiration. In addition, recognition is accorded to several generations of physiotherapy students from Dalhousie University whose enthusiasm and creativity ensured the ongoing development of a relevant physiotherapy service for this unique community-based group.

Contents

1 | Introduction

George I. Turnbull

When the term *Parkinson's disease* (PD) is used, there is a tendency to visualize a disabled individual with a typical flexed posture, immobile features, and a tremor that is most pronounced in the hands.[1] The gait pattern is the typical "marche à petits pas" and the subject is prone to getting "stuck" at inopportune times.[2] Unfortunately, the symptoms just described are those of a person only in the later stages of the disease. A person with PD can also appear completely normal and demonstrate no disability, as is the case in the early stages of the disorder or while the disease is controlled by medication. The reason for making this observation is to allow the physical therapist to examine his or her own perception of the disease. The first scenario described above is the one more likely to be familiar, because by the time of referral for physical therapy, the PD patient has often reached the later stages of the disease. To be effective in managing PD physical therapists will probably need to change this perception of the typical PD patient.

Physical therapy was developed initially as a method for treating patients with orthopedic-type injuries.[3] The system of physical therapy that has evolved as a result of this includes assessing and treating a patient for specific periods (30-minute blocks of time or multiples thereof), with the frequency of these sessions dependent on the severity of the symptoms. For example, a patient with acute back symptoms may initially be treated on a daily basis, with the frequency of treatment diminishing as the patient's symptoms improve. The assumption underlying this philosophy is that the patient is first seen while symptoms are acute, with improvement expected in subsequent visits. The "disability"-to-"normality" mindset is satisfying to both therapist and patient and reinforces the notion of "cure" as the ultimate objective of care. This "orthopedic" paradigm is probably appropriate for patients with orthopedic-type injuries and has been adopted by institutions and insurance agencies as the norm for the practice of physical therapy. Unfortunately, this philosophy of physical therapy practice has spilled over into other parts of the profession,

1

including the area of neurologic rehabilitation, where it appears to be inappropriate in view of the bodies of knowledge of how the central nervous system adapts to injury or pathology and that concerned with the retraining of movement. In addition to this, many neurologic conditions are degenerative, necessitating a departure from the "cure" mentality. It appears to be essential that physical therapists working in the area of neurologic rehabilitation reconsider some of the assumptions that dictate treatment scheduling, including the limitations imposed by insurance and institutional considerations. The physical therapy management of PD is an example of the inadequacy of the current paradigm.

As David King aptly points out in Chapter 2 of this book, PD, unlike any other neurologic condition, has been significantly altered in terms of its clinical progression by the development of effective medications. As a result of the success of these drugs, the functional capacity of the patient is prolonged for many years. Given the modus operandus of physical therapy in the current healthcare system, intervention is typically undertaken when the patient begins to experience significant functional difficulty. It is then that referral to the physical therapist occurs for the first time. At this stage the patient may have had PD for 7 to 10 years. The real reason for the referral is that medical science has exhausted its options and physical therapy is used in the hope that minor functional gains can be made to facilitate the care of the patient. Upon examination, however, this reactive role of the physical therapist is less than adequate, because the therapist possesses no magical restorative powers. All that can be done for the patient at this stage of the disease is to analyze problems and suggest more efficient motor strategies or "tricks" to enhance function, propose a more ergonomically sound living environment, and counsel caregivers about such matters as assisted transfers, feeding, speech, and how to deal with specific functional deficiencies. In other words, the role of the physical therapist is to help the patient adapt to diminishing functional capabilities. Although these objectives are relevant and helpful, the effectiveness of the therapist in working toward them is often hampered by the debilitated state of the patient. Exercise tolerance is diminished, posture is poor, and injuries may have occurred through such accidents as falls. The patient may also be suffering from nutritional deficiencies, which will further complicate the picture. Before any useful management can begin, the therapist has a great deal to do in attempts to rectify this "disuse" situation. Clearly, intervention has taken place too late for physical therapy to stand any chance of being successful. In this paradigm, physical therapy is probably ineffective—a conclusion that is not that surprising when it is carefully analyzed. Consequently, there appears to be a need to re-examine the role of the physical therapist in the management of the patient with PD, particularly with regard to the reactive nature of the approach to such therapy, which should be replaced by a much more proactive philosophy. It is one purpose of this book to propose some options so that this redefinition can take place.

Before the development of L-dopa, the physical therapist often felt a sense of helplessness and frustration at the appearance of a PD patient on the referral list. Physical therapeutic methods included attempts at treating the classic clinical triad of bradykinesia, rigidity, and tremor. Other procedures included massage and relaxation techniques to reduce rigidity, limit postural deformities, and improve the patient's lung function.[4] Attention was given to gait "re-education," often through the use of visual cues[5] and rhythmical movements to counteract "freezing".[6] Techniques such as warm baths, massage, and hydrotherapy were also advocated.[7] Although referral was often made with the objective of treating later-stage complications such as chest infections or pressure sores, the foregoing practices were essentially aimed at minimizing the effect of the inevitable disability. Then, in 1971, a group of South African physical therapists reported an increased referral of patients with PD[8] as the result of the advent of L-dopa. Seizing this challenge, these therapists treated the patients vigorously, using rhythmic activities performed on mats to reduce rigidity; rocking techniques; modified procedures derived from the Knott and Voss, Rood, and Temple Fay approaches; the encouragement of truncal rotation to assist gait; and the treatment of facial expression and lung function. Individual treatment sessions were combined with group instruction in home-exercise routines. The author of the South African report postulated that physical therapy in conjunction with L-dopa therapy enhanced patient progress. Implied in her statement was the philosophy that the objective of physical therapy was to "restore" function.

The citation of this 1971 work is not meant to be critical of these therapists, who are instead to be commended for adopting an innovative program at a critical period in history and for sharing their experiences through publication. Their work is cited here to illustrate the assumption that physical therapy in PD is effective through some process yet to be understood. The physical therapist must accept that there is no evidence for the contention that physical therapy as currently employed has any effect on the pathology of PD, therefore the sensible first step for physical therapists to take in developing an effective approach to the management of PD is to assume the null hypothesis in terms of influencing the disease itself. In fact, in 1981, Gibberd et al.[9] found in a controlled study that physical therapy was ineffective against PD itself. However, there is also the need to resist the temptation to dismiss physiotherapy as a treatment option for patients with PD. I can vividly recall the indignation of my students when they returned from a lecture on PD in which a prominent neurologist (and author of a chapter in this book) stated that the disease was not conducive to physical therapy. Given the evidence, his statement was correct. What the profession of physical therapy must now do is to consider realistically its role in the treatment of this difficult disorder and to resist the tempting contention that it can ameliorate the disease itself. Because it is unlikely that this can be done, fresh attitudes and perspectives must be developed.

Another purpose of this book is to consider the work of others, some in disciplines other than physical therapy, and to develop a framework for treatment of the patient with PD that is realistic and sensible in the light of new knowledge. With the advent of new methods of administering L-dopa, such as slow-release medications now available, the promising role of bromocriptine, and the encouraging though still controversial research relating to Deprenyl (selegiline hydrochloride), the redefinition of the role of physical therapy is becoming a priority. This becomes even more urgent should the research on transplantation of dopamine-producing tissues, as described in the chapter by Fine and Rasmusson, prove effective and ethically acceptable. It is hoped that the content of this book will stimulate further innovation as well as providing some immediate solutions to treatment of the PD patient. In addition, it will be necessary to test both current and future physical therapy procedures so that the PD population is served in a manner that truly provides it with help. Before these objectives of physical therapy can be attained, it is necessary to question many of the assumptions on which the profession functions.

Physical therapists encounter a number of neurologic conditions that are progressive. Multiple sclerosis, Huntington's disease, and amytrophic lateral sclerosis are examples. As is the case with PD, physical therapy for these disorders is not clearly defined. However, there are models from which a logical approach to the care of the PD patient can be developed. Figure 1-1 compares the "cure"-oriented model with that of a model that could be used in the management of any patient with a progressive disorder of the central nervous system. In addition, the model that is often now adopted for the care of the PD patient is shown. This latter profile is based on the premise that medication will initially restore all function. Indeed, the patient in this phase of PD appears completely normal but may develop symptoms as the medication wears off. Only later, when the medication becomes less effective or unpredictable and the patient begins to suffer loss of functional ability, will the physical therapist be asked to intervene. By this time, the patient has developed the disuse syndrome mentioned earlier, which significantly complicates the effectiveness of the physical therapist. As a result, this framework for physical therapy management of PD is unsatisfactory. The "cure" framework is also inappropriate because it must be accepted that with time, the patient will deteriorate to a point at which he or she will be unable to function. This leaves the "progressive" paradigm for managing PD. Clearly, the emphasis of care will change as the patient's condition deteriorates. In fact, the "progressive" model is almost rehabilitation in reverse, in that the patient begins therapy in a functionally capable state and the physical therapist's job is to keep the patient in an optimal condition for as long as possible.[10] This could be done by improving the patient's condition from a cardiovascular viewpoint as well as by working on muscle function, joint flexibility, gait, and balance. Hogan et al[11] have shown that normal elderly people can preserve function over time by undertaking general exercises on a twice weekly basis. In the same study, the subjects' balance and muscle strength both actually improved, but only after a prolonged period of exercise.[12] Because the types of difficulties experienced by the PD patient as the condition progresses can be predicted in a general sense, it should be possible to adapt a general exercise program to include measures specifically directed at preventing these difficulties. It is critical, however, that such a program be initiated as soon as possible after the condition is diagnosed, and before the musculoskeletal changes and motor characteristics related to PD become entrenched.

"CURE" PARADIGM

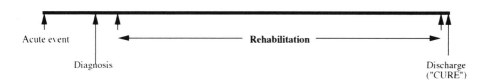

CURRENT PARKINSON'S PARADIGM

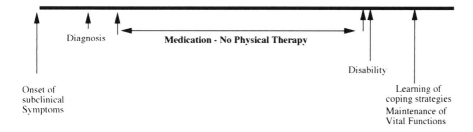

"PROGRESSIVE" PARADIGM

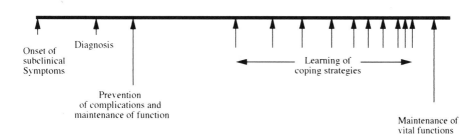

Fig. 1-1. Three models for physical therapy management: (1) the cure model; (2) the model frequently used to manage patients with Parkinson's disease; and (3) the progressive model.

In addition to this preventive treatment strategy, a number of other components of a physical therapy program for PD require attention before such a plan would work. Careful monitoring and documentation of the results of that monitoring appear essential. The objective of this component of care is to be able to track the functional profile of the patient over time, so that the exercise program can be adjusted rapidly in response to the particular way in which the disease is affecting a given patient. For example, Melnick[13] has proposed the use of the evaluation format published by Endo Laboratories. This subjective evaluation allows the patient to be scored on a four-point scale in 10 categories that are critical in PD. These 10 categories are bradykinesia of the hands, rigidity, posture, upper-extremity swing, gait, tremor, facial expression, seborrhea, speech, and self-care. The cumulative point total in the evaluation permits each patient to be classified into three "disability" categories. These are "Early Illness," "Moderate Disability," and "Severe or Advanced Disease." The real value of this system, however, is that it permits determination of the areas in which dysfunction is most pronounced. This permits the physical therapist to attend to priorities as they arise, and to ensure that the treatment provided to a given patient targets the specific symptoms of PD as it has affected that patient. Although more difficult to obtain, objective testing measures are also desirable. The advantage of including quantitative assessment of each patient is that it minimizes the element of bias or error that can enter into the assessment process. Regular measures of balance and gait would seem to be useful in monitoring change over time. Although many objective systems for evaluating gait are expensive and thus beyond the reach of many physical therapists, there are practical and economically acceptable methods available. These methods are described by Wall in Chapter 5 of this book.

A third component that seems to be essential in considering a new paradigm for the management of PD is an educational element. This role could easily fall into the province of the physical therapist because, in recent years, physical therapy programs have increasingly adopted the coverage of human learning and educational methods as part of their curricula.[14] This background, together with a knowledge of functional anatomy and applied biomechanics, a sound knowledge of the progression of the disease and its symptoms, and how all of this affects function puts the physical therapist in an ideal position to educate both the patient and other nonprofessional caregivers in a meaningful way. The integration of this educational component into an overall package of patient management will be described in Chapter 7 of this book, by Turnbull.

Given that a multifaceted physical therapy program is being suggested as a viable way to manage patients with PD, it is vital that the physical therapist fully appreciate more than just the musculoskeletal and motor aspects of this disorder. An understanding of the cognitive and of the direct and indirect psychological manifestations of the disease will enhance the role of the physical therapist when treating and interacting with the patient. When it is considered that the physical therapist will be dealing with such concepts as motivation, communication, and education, the "non-locomotor" aspects of PD become significant. It is not being proposed that the physical therapist attempt to treat these latter manifestations of PD, because there are healthcare professionals who are better prepared for this aspect of care. However, the type of interaction that is being proposed to allow this model of physical therapy to work demands knowledge of the psychological or affective effects of PD. Chapter 6 of this book, by Fisk and Doble, is designed to meet this objective.

In concluding this introductory chapter, it seems high time to reconsider the role of physical therapy in the management of the patient with PD. There is also a need to refashion the structure and context of the greater part of physical therapy when dealing with this disorder. Although it appears highly unlikely that physical therapy can effect a change in the course of the disease process, its emphasis in the management of PD can be preventive, while also ensuring that the patient reaches and maintains full potential from a "fitness" viewpoint. Any deficiencies caused by the progression of PD would be detected and dealt with promptly by adjusting the exercise program so that the patient could relearn the deteriorating motor skills. According to Chapter 4 of this book, by Stelmach and Phillips, this is an attainable objective. However, for this strategy to be effective, methods of assessment that effectively detect change must be included and frequently applied. In addition to the system of monitoring already mentioned, Chapter 5, by Wall, and Chapter 8 by Sharpe, offer further suggestions in this regard.

Although this discussion has advocated the proactive philosophy of physical therapy for PD, there is still a place for the use of physical therapy procedures for the management of specific motor manifestations of the disease. In addition to describing these procedures, Chapter 9, by Schenkman, also addresses the context in which these techniques may be applied for maximum benefit.

The long-term nature of the care in PD also makes critically important the structure needed to permit achieving objectives described above. Economy of time and costs, patient motivation, and compliance with long-term exercise programs and educational requirements, together with the need of each patient to identify and solve problems with others who share the same concerns, appear to be essential ingredients. It is up to the physical therapy community to work with PD patients and nonprofessional caregivers, as well as other relevant healthcare professionals, to develop solutions to these problems. It is hoped that this book will help physical therapists to achieve these objectives.

REFERENCES

1. Gibberd FB: The clinical findings and pathology in Parkinson's disease. Physiotherapy 72:333, 1986
2. Handford F: Parkinson's disease: introduction. Physiotherapy 72:332, 1986
3. Young PH: A short history of the C.S.P. Physiotherapy 56:271, 1969
4. Cailliet R: Rehabilitation in Parkinsonism. In Licht S (ed): Rehabilitation and Medicine. Licht, New Haven, Connecticut, 1968
5. Martin JP: Locomotion and the basal ganglia. In Martin JP (ed): The Basal Ganglia and Posture. JB Lippincott, Philadelphia, 1967
6. Ball JM: Demonstration of the traditional approach in the treatment of a patient with Parkinsonism. Am J Phys Med 46:1034, 1967
7. Rusk HA: Rehabilitation Medicine. 3rd Ed. CV Mosby, St. Louis, 1971
8. Irwin-Carruthers SH: An approach to physiotherapy for the patient with Parkinson's disease. S Afr J Physiother 25:5, 1971
9. Gibberd FB, Page NGR, Spender KM, Kinnear E, Hawksworth JB: Controlled trial

of physiotherapy and occupational therapy for Parkinson's disease. BMJ 282:1196, 1981

10. Kinnear E: Long Term management of Parkinson's disease. Physiotherapy 72:340, 1986
11. Hogan DB, Wall JC, Beresford P et al: The effects of an exercise program on parameters of balance and gait in the elderly. In preparation
12. Turnbull GI, Wall JC, Hogan DB, Fox RA: The effects of a general exercise programme on the ability of elderly women to control postural responses. Physiother Can 43(Suppl 4):17, 1991
13. Melnick ME: Basal ganglia disorders. In Umphred DA (ed): Neurological Rehabilitation. CV Mosby, St. Louis, 1990
14. Canadian Physiotherapy Association: Recommended Core Curriculum for Physiotherapy Education Programmes. Canadian Physiotherapy Association, Toronto, 1986

2 | Diagnosis, Pharmacology, and Medical Management

Drug Management

David B. King

Parkinson's disease (PD) opened new vistas for neurologic therapeutics. It was the first degenerative disease to be successfully managed and dimly understood. While time has tempered the initial enthusiasm about its successful management, it is clear that current methods of managing PD make a significant contribution to the patient's quality of life.

DEFINITIONS

Parkinson's disease is a disorder of unknown etiology involving certain pigmented nuclei of the brain stem, particularly the substantia nigra and pars compacta, which always show cell loss and commonly also exhibit intracytoplasmic inclusions called Lewy bodies.

Parkinson's syndrome, or parkinsonism, manifests the clinical features of PD, including tremor, rigidity, bradykinesia, and postural abnormalities, but differs pathologically and therapeutically from the disease.

PATHOPHYSIOLOGY

The destruction of the substantia nigra results in a striatal depletion of the neurotransmitter dopamine. As a result, acetylcholine becomes the dominant transmitter in the striatum. The treatment of PD attempts to correct this imbalance, ignoring the other transmitters whose functions remain unknown.

Clearly, various pathologies may assault and destroy the black nucleus, leaving in their wake the parkinsonian syndrome. Infections, vasculopathies,

9

drugs, chemicals, genetic deficiencies, and certain structural diseases are among these. The etiology of PD remains mysterious.

Classically, the great 1918 influenza epidemic and its cerebral concomitant, encephalitis lethargica, produced a cohort of parkinsonian patients, particularized by other movement disorders and oculogyric crisis. The virus left gliosis and tangled microtubular structures throughout the brain stem nuclei and the striatum. Rarely, other pathogens, such as the spirochete of syphilis, other encephalopathic viruses, and the viroids of Creutzfeldt-Jakob disease produce parkinsonism.

Bilateral infarctions of the basal ganglia, alone or as part of the multiinfarct state, produce parkinsonism as a component of a more diffuse cerebral illness.

Most secondary parkinsonism stems from the aggressive use of psychiatric medications of the dopamine-depleting or dopamine-blocking variety. Phenothiazines, thioxanthines, and butyrophenones are the chief offenders. Metaclopramide, valuable in gastrointestinal medicine, is often a forgotten culprit. Parkinsonism may smolder on for months after the offending agents are stopped.

Manganese miners, after several months exposure to manganese ore, may manifest parkinsonism superimposed on an encephalopathy. Carbon disulfide, carbon monoxide, and cyanide may all produce a contaminated parkinsonism. Recently a byproduct of meperidine manufacture, MPTP, caused a rather pure parkinsonian syndrome in humans and primates. Small gaggles of conscientious drug abusers, attempting to manufacture meperidine in their basement laboratories, produced instead its toxic congener, which targeted the cells in the substantia nigra, causing an acute to subacute parkinsonian syndrome. This provided a dramatic model of the disease, and the abusers a poor prognosis. The syndrome in primates may be prevented by a monoamine oxidase-B (MAO-B) inhibitor, selegiline (Deprenyl), which prevents the breakdown of MPTP to MPP+.

Certain uncommon metabolic diseases may deceive the unwary. Wilson's disease, an autosomal recessive disease, deposits copper in the brain, cornea, liver, and kidney. Parkinsonism is distinctly in its repertoire. Multiple bouts of hepatic encephalopathy, among drinkers of alcohol, produce hepatocerebral degeneration in which parkinsonism complicates dementia, ataxia, and upper-motor-neuron findings. A complex disorder of iron metabolism in children can produce the Hallervorden-Spatz syndrome. Its rarity and time preclude a detailed description of this condition. Calcification in the basal ganglia can be confusing, producing no or significant pathology. It obviously depends on the site of calcium deposition.

Tumors, hydrocephalus, and pugilistic encephalopathy may all produce syndromes of which parkinsonism is at least a part.

A large group of diseases of the degenerative variety masquerade as PD. Often, their true nature is only revealed when the patient fails to respond to L-dopa. The prognosis is uniformly poor. Associated neurologic features, magnetic resonance imaging (MRI), and computed tomography (CT) have allowed their more accurate clinical differentiation.

Parkinson's disease itself is viewed primarily as a disease of certain brain stem nuclei, in particular the substantia nigra. Although its cause is unknown, current speculation suggests a toxin. It is further supposed that the death of cells in the substantia nigra, whatever the primary cause, is secondary to an oxidative process acting on the walls of organelles and cells. This oxidation may arise from the byproducts of dopamine catabolism through MAO-B.

TREATMENT

Medications designed to prevent the progress of PD are vitamin E and selegiline (Deprenyl). Medications designed to redress the striatal imbalance caused by PD are (1) L-dopa (Sinemet); (2) amantidine (Symmetril); (3) bromocriptine (Parlodel); (4) apomorphine; (5) other dopaminergic analogues; and (6) anticholinergics.

MANAGEMENT

Immediately after being diagnosed as having PD, the patient should probably be started on selegiline in the fixed dose of 5 mg given in the morning and again at noon. This dose is adequate to block all MAO-B in the central nervous system (CNS), thereby preventing the formation of superoxides, preserving cellular integrity, and arresting the disease process. A recent study[1] suggested that selegeline was doing exactly that and not influencing the symptoms of the disease. There is certainly evidence to the contrary. This author believes there are design faults in the study that make its conclusions suspect.

Selegiline has few side effects, and despite reservations, it should therefore be employed in making the diagnosis of PD. Its stimulant properties require doses confined to the first half of the day. Amphetamine and methamphetamine are products of selegiline metabolism. Presumably because the amounts of amphetamine are relatively small, addiction has not been described.

Despite the attractive oxidative theory of the cause of PD, the DATATOP study provides no support for the use of vitamin E in the disease.

Some 2 years or less after the diagnosis of PD is made, selegiline becomes ineffective and additional therapy is required. Bromocriptine may be the first choice. As a dopaminergic analogue, it acts postsynaptically by stimulating the denervated striatal cells. At lower doses it may work presynaptically to block dopaminergic nerve endings, thereby stimulating the production of more dopamine. It is started at a low dose and increased slowly to symptomatic benefit, with doses that in most instances should not exceed 30 mg/day. Postural hypotension will be aggravated by bromocriptine. If there is any degree of dementia the drug is better avoided, thereby preventing a delirium that may take several days to resolve after cessation of therapy. Bromocriptine causes gastrointestinal distress, but this is usually mild and dealt with easily. The drug is started (as Parlodel) at 2.5 mg/day and increased by 2.5 mg/day/week, with an expected beneficial response at about 20 mg, although a dose as high as 30 mg is sometimes needed. Certain authorities believe that patients can be maintained on doses as low as 2.5 mg t.i.d., with benefits equal to those at higher doses. This is true in mild to moderate PD, because of the survival of at least some substantia nigra cells. More advanced disease requires higher doses, if tolerated, to stimulate the striatum. Doses exceeding 30 mg/day are sometimes used. The adverse effects of postural hypotension, nausea, and confusion with bromocriptine become more prominent at such doses.

After about 1 to 2 years on this therapy, the patient will note a loss of effectiveness but seldom abnormal movements. L-dopa, in the form of Sinemet, may be added to the bromocriptine. Sinemet is started at about 100 mg/day, Sinemet 100/25 being a convenient preparation. After two 100-mg increments, 100 mg at four day intervals, the patient should be followed for at least 2 months before considering a change. It is not unusual to exceed 800 mg/day of L-dopa. Frequently, lower doses will suffice. What is needed is the lowest dose that will correct the patient's complaints rather than restore a state of normality. Symptoms, not signs, should be treated. Function is more important than cosmetics.

Tremor may increase at about this time, or it may never have been fully responsive to bromocriptine or L-dopa. Tremor is not infrequently the patient's main complaint, more because of embarrassment than functional loss.

For either reason, the tremor may demand treatment. Often, it fails to respond to any treatment agent. Anticholinergics, such as benztropine mesylate, may prove helpful. Benztropine mesylate may be started at 2 mg b.i.d. and increased very slowly, though doses much above 6 mg daily are rarely tolerated because of the typical cholinergic side effects of dry mouth, blurred vision, constipation, urinary retention, and confusion. If Benztropine mesylate fails or is not tolerated, clonazepam (Rivotril) may be used in doses up to 6 mg daily. Drowsiness, particularly at higher doses, limits its usefulness. Rarely propranolol will help, although theoretically it should not. Perhaps it reduces anxiety and thereby attenuates tremor.

Parkinson's disease continues to progress. After another year or two the patient will again notice increasing wearing-off of each dose and the gradual development of abnormal movements or dyskinesias. These are said to be less if the patient is on low doses of L-dopa. If the dyskinesias are mild, the patient's drug regimen should be maintained. If they are moderate and management is required, a course of amantidine at 100 mg b.i.d. or t.i.d. may be tried with simultaneous reduction in the dosage of L-dopa. The main side effects are livedo reticularis, and in patients predisposed to them, seizures. There is salt retention with this drug, and caution should be exercised if the patient has a history of congestive heart failure. Amantidine, if helpful at all, tends not to provide benefits for more than 6 months, probably because of the induction of tachyphylaxis.

As the abnormal movements increase in intensity, it is usually necessary to increase the dosing frequency of both bromocriptine and L-dopa. The frequency probably can be increased to five times per day. Above that frequency, in most patients, the fluctuation of performance will occur at unpredictable times. It is rational at this point to reduce the number of daily doses, allowing the patient more predictable off-drug periods so that the patient can arrange an appropriate daily schedule.

If the fluctuations continue to be severe and are unresponsive to an increasing dose frequency or to modifications of the ratio of L-dopa to bromocriptine, then it is possible to use Sinemet-CR 200/50, a sustained release form of L-dopa. One can expect benefits for a time, but the continued advance of the disease with the loss of cells in the substantia nigra that are capable of converting L-dopa to dopamine, and presumably the irregular L-dopa-to-dopamine conversion metabolism of cells in the striatum, lead to failure of a sustained response to L-dopa even in this formulation.

Unfortunately, the complication of dementia may supervene. It then becomes necessary to reduce the dosage of the medications being used to treat the disease. Usually the anticholinergic is reduced first, followed by bromocriptine and L-dopa. The patient's mental status must take priority over the motor abnormalities.

Some seven years after the onset of PD, the patient is no longer responsive to therapy. This is particularly the case when the patient is demented. Management at this stage is temporizing and more dependent on family support and nursing care.

If the patient is not demented and the motor abnormalities are severe, there are still some possible therapeutic strategies, but most are available in specialized centers. I will not discuss these in detail, but simply list them:

1. Subcutaneous apomorphine
2. Gastrostomy administered L-dopa
3. Fetal mesencephalic transplants
4. Autologous adrenal transplants
5. Transdermal dopaminergic analogues

CONCLUSIONS

Current treatment may be expected to maintain parkinsonian patients in optimum health for about 7 years. After that there are increasing difficulties, culminating in dementia with a consequent shift to nursing rather than medical management.

Long-Term Care

Roy A. Fox

In the practice of geriatric medicine, patients are seen with both Parkinson's disease (PD) and parkinsonism, as defined in the first part of this chapter. Some patients are presenting for the first time, and for the most part they need to be treated in the same way as younger patients and with medications as discussed. With the frail elderly who have interacting physical, mental, and social problems, the approach to medication needs to be modified. This will be discussed. In addition, many patients are seen who have had PD for a long time; these individuals are usually experiencing side effects and often aggravation of other problems. Such patients, often with end-stage disease, need careful adjustment of their medications, and frequently require discontinuation of many of their medications. In this group of patients, other aspects of care become of greater importance, and the role of nursing, physiotherapy, occupational therapy, and social work needs to be stressed.

DRUG THERAPY IN OLD AGE

With advancing age, each of us is exposed to the deleterious effects of aging processes as well as a variety of disease processes. The net effect is decreasing reserve and increasing susceptibility to stressors. In the population of frail elderly persons, these effects are most pronounced, and culminate in the frailty itself with its associated risk of dysfunction and of being admitted to an institution. Parkinson's disease may strike anyone at any time, although it becomes increasingly common with advancing age. The disease may occur in the setting of an otherwise healthy host or in one who is already burdened with disease and dysfunctional. But old age and wellness represent a continuum from those persons who are fully functional and independent to those who are dysfunctional in multiple areas and dependent, and there are individuals who remain relatively well and independent provided there are no stressors. These could be referred to as *prefrail* persons. Parkinson's disease represents an additional, very significant burden to such people, and they become extremely vulnerable to sudden deterioration with additional stress, and to the side effects of drugs. In fact, iatrogenic disease from misplaced enthusiasm in the use of drugs leads to severe dysfunction in such patients. The proportion of these individuals increases with advancing age, and may be difficult to predict before therapy. For this reason drug therapy in old age should be approached with caution, and should be modified in all but overtly healthy older persons.

The same drugs are to be used as in younger patients, but the dosage should be modified. Selegiline should be started at half the usual dose, with 5 mg in the morning or, in the obviously frail, 2.5 mg once a day. The dosage should be increased only if the patient is free of side effects that lead to dysfunction. This drug should be reserved for the patient with newly diagnosed PD.

For the patient who is symptomatic with rigidity, bradykinesia, or tremor, the drug of choice is L-dopa. For most patients the regimen already described is appropriate, although in the frail and those individuals with any evidence of cognitive decline it is wise to begin with half the usual dose, or half of a 100/25 tablet of Sinemet, increasing to two halves in 4 days and to three halves 4 days later. If all is well, with no significant side effects, the morning dose can be increased to a full tablet and then increased every 4 days until acceptable symptomatic relief is obtained. Although this is slow, it is a much safer approach to therapy.

The most important side effects of drug therapy for PD in the frail and cognitively impaired elderly are related to cognitive dysfunction. Increasing cognitive impairment may occur, which implies that such patients need to be carefully monitored, with repeated assessment of their cognitive state. There may be associated hallucinations or delusions, and delirium can be precipitated quite easily in many of these patients. Correct management is to discontinue the drug until all symptoms are cleared, attend to any other likely precipitants of delirium, and then carefully reintroduce the medication and proceed very slowly with any increase in dosage. Bromocriptine is even more likely to produce these side effects in the frail elderly, and can therefore rarely be utilized. If it is necessary to try this drug because of other side effects of L-dopa, then the regimen described is appropriate. Older patients can usually be controlled on lower doses than younger patients, and frequently a dosage level of 5 mg t.i.d. is adequate.

Many older patients have coincident atherosclerosis, ischemic heart disease, and hypertension. Antiparkinsonian medication may also precipitate orthostatic hypotension. Patients with PD are predisposed to this, and the addition of a medication such as L-dopa or bromocriptine is sufficient to precipitate significant hypotension. This in turn may result in a fall and severe injury or dysfunction. All patients need to be carefully monitored and need to have their recumbent and standing blood pressures measured at each visit, with questions asked about the onset of dizziness or lightheadedness on first standing. When these patients are on multiple drugs they should undergo comprehensive geriatric assessment and modification of their drug regimen. When antiparkinsonian drugs are necessary to maintain adequate function, other drugs that are not lifesaving or even life enhancing can be discontinued or modified.

Anticholinergic drugs such as benztropine mesylate can rarely be tolerated by the frail elderly because of the risk of hallucinations, the precipitation of delirium, and severe dysfunction.

Other drug side effects are similar in all age groups and are managed in the usual way.

COMPREHENSIVE GERIATRIC ASSESSMENT

To determine the nature of the PD patient's problems and the possible negative impact of medications, it is essential to perform what is referred to as a comprehensive geriatric assessment (CGA). Only in this way will a full picture of the patient's condition be obtained. A physician can collect most of the information, but a CGA is best done by a full healthcare team, which includes a geriatrician, nurse, social worker, occupational therapist, and physiotherapist. Such a team usually functions within a geriatric day hospital, specialized ambulatory care facility, or patient geriatric evaluation and management (GEM) unit. The team also requires access to other health professionals such as a dietitian, psychologist, or speech pathologist. Experience has shown that frail elderly persons do better in such settings and with complete assessments. Only in this way can the correct therapy for the multiple, interacting problems of the elderly PD patient be achieved. The assessment is far reaching and goes beyond what is usually considered to be part of the management of PD. Experience has shown that the format described in Table 2-1 is appropriate.

With a CGA, each area of possible dysfunction can be identified. The heading of Mental Status incorporates the patient's cognitive abilities, intellectual function, and memory. In order to diagnose or confirm the presence of intellectual dysfunction, an appropriate history-taking is required. The members of the healthcare team should ask about the patient's everyday function and whether the spouse or significant other has noted any decline in function. Questions should be asked about the patient's ability to manage financial affairs, about memory lapses, and whether there are any behavioral changes. Often the spouse will express concerns about the patient's declining abilities before the physician suspects that there is any problem. An appropriate screening tool would be a simple scale of instrumental activities of daily living, such as that of Lawton.[3] If dysfunction is suspected, then administration of a mini-mental

Table 2-1. Comprehensive Geriatric Assessment

Functional Assessment	
1. Mental state	
2. Emotional	
3. Communication	
4. Mobility	
5. Balance (history of falls)	
6. Bowel function	
7. Urinary function	
8. Nutrition	
9. Daily activities	
10. Social	

Pathophysiologic Problems	Associated medications
1–10 list active problems	Identify each drug, dose and timing (prescription and over-the-counter). Each drug must have an associated problem.

status examination[4] would be appropriate. If cognitive impairment is confirmed, it is important for the physician to determine the likely etiology. If dementia is diagnosed, as it is in about 14 percent to 20 percent of patients with PD,[5] then it is the responsibility of the physician and members of the healthcare team to ensure that the patient is at optimal function, since this has a major bearing on the quality of life of both the patient and the care providers. Dementia is a major risk factor for delirium, indicating that such patients have very limited reserve in cognitive function. Patients with PD may present for the first time with delirium at the time of hospitalization or surgery. This is often secondary to medications, and may be the first sign of cognitive decline.[6] Note should be made of any particular areas of behavioral disturbance that need modification. Perhaps the most significant area of inquiry is into management of medications. Many PD patients are on multiple medications, and their understanding and whether they are conforming to the prescribed regimen need to be determined. When it is determined that there is a problem, the drug regimen requires simplification, and supervision must often be handed over to a family member or professional.

Under the heading of *Emotional,* the mood of the patient is carefully assessed to determine if depression is a problem. This is a common problem in old age, and is certainly more common in association with PD.[7] It may result in significant cognitive impairment, and treatment of the depression will therefore result in improvement of cognitive function and sometimes a return to normal. The patient's personality needs to be determined, as do the patient's health attitudes, which will have a significant bearing on rehabilitation and compliance with therapy.

Under the heading of *Communication,* difficulties with vision, hearing, or speech are determined. In this context many patients with PD have speech problems and will benefit from a formal assessment and ongoing therapy from a speech pathologist.

Mobility is an ongoing problem with all PD patients. Information about it can be gathered by the administration of an instrument such as Barthel's Index. In this way the nature of the mobility problem and its impact on the patient's daily life and care provision can be determined. The patient needs careful assessment by a physiotherapist skilled in the care of patients with PD. In the earlier stages of the disease the physiotherapist can help with teaching the patient techniques to reduce rigidity and to help initiate movement. As the disease progresses, care providers can also be trained to help the patient overcome blocks and instances of freezing during movement. Ongoing assessment and the maintenance of an objective measurement of ability to perform simple tasks is crucial. As part of this, each patient can perform the Get up and Go test,[8,9] which is timed. In this way, objective information on decline and also improvement with rehabilitation can be checked.

The physiotherapist, together with the occupational therapist, will also need to be involved in the assessment of *Balance:* sitting, standing, and dynamic. Dynamic balance is the first to deteriorate in PD. Falling becomes a major problem with PD. Maintaining flexibility and maintaining muscle strength by a

Table 2-2. Mobility and Balance Care

Stage	Professional	Role	Outcome
All	Physiotherapy	Exercise program; relaxation	Flexibility; improve strength
At diagnosis	Physiotherapy	Education	Improve understanding
Late	Physiotherapy	Assessment; prescription of aids	Improve mobility Improve balance Reduce risks
Late	Occupational therapy	Assessment; prescription	Enhance balance
Advanced	Physiotherapy	Assessment	Modify rigidity
Advanced	Occupational therapy	Home/ environmental Assessment/ prescription	Modify falls Improve safety; reduce risk of serious injury

regular exercise program helps enormously in minimizing deterioration. However, deterioration is inevitable. A time comes when balance and walking aids are required. It is at this point that the skill and experience of the physiotherapist are crucial. Many PD patients are less safe with a regular cane, since it is often treated as an obstacle and may precipitate falls. The same holds true for regular walkers; although these are beneficial in some patients, in those with perceptual problems or who are dyspraxic with impaired judgement, they increase risk rather than enhance safety. Such patients may benefit from the provision of a wheeled walker, but many are best without any aid. When mobility or balance cannot be improved, one is left with a situation in which much counselling is required, and if continuing mobility, despite its risks, is decided upon by the family and the patient, then environmental assessment is essential. The occupational therapist should assess the patient's home environment and offer advice in improving safety and reducing the risk of environmentally induced falls. In advanced stages of the disease, safety equipment can be recommended to the patient that might reduce the risk or impact of serious injury. Examples of this include modified helmets or limb protectors (Table 2-2).

The assessment of *Bowel Function* may not seem relevant in this setting, but is extremely important in the elderly patient, particularly the frail elderly. Many patients with PD have bowel dysfunction, and severe constipation is a common problem that may result in impaction with pseudo-obstruction or fecal incontinence. The physician needs to determine the patient's usual bowel habit and any problems. The physician, nurse, and dietician can help PD patients to better manage their bowels and overcome their difficulties without resorting to the extensive use of purgatives. Improved function will often lead to an enhanced feeling of well being, improved cognitive function, and an all-around improvement in the patient. This is often of major significance in the patient with advanced disease.

Urinary Function also needs careful evaluation. Urinary incontinence is a common problem among the frail elderly, and should be asked about. If present, it must be assessed by the physician and nurse. The pattern of incontinence will provide important clues about its cause. Patients with advanced PD may have coincident problems such as detrusor instability, or the incontinence may be directly related to PD or its treatment. In advanced disease the patient may be unable to reach a toilet in time, despite being aware of a full bladder and the need to go to a toilet. If this is determined to be the case, then the patient may be helped by exercises to improve flexibility and mobility. Occupational therapy may be able to help by modification of clothing when dexterity is limited. Environmental modification may also be of benefit if toilet access can be improved. Drug review may reveal medications that are increasing urine flow (such as diuretics) or reducing bladder tone (such as antidepressants or tranquilizers), thus promoting urine retention with overflow. Drug modification may help. If specific problems are identified, the prescription of certain drugs, such as an anticholinergic, may help with detrusor instability.

A significant proportion of frail elderly persons have nutritional problems, particularly those with some degree of cognitive impairment and who live alone. Assessment of *Nutrition* is of paramount importance. If it becomes apparent that impaired nutrition is a problem, then careful assessment should reveal the reasons. Patients with PD who live alone may have difficulty with food preparation or with food acquisition and meal planning. This will only be determined by an occupational therapeutic assessment and, if necessary, by kitchen and meal planning assessments. Training can be provided, but very often, provision of help will be required, such as enlisting the help of homemakers or "meals on wheels." As the disease progresses, more care with food preparation is required to enable patients to masticate their food and swallow it. A point will be reached at which the patient will require help with feeding. Before this stage is reached, the occupational therapist will be able to recommend modification of utensils to help the impaired patient.

Under the heading of *Daily Activities,* any problem that the patient is having in routine daily tasks is noted. A convenient way to determine this is to administer instruments such as Barthel's Index[10] plus a scale for instrumental activities of daily living.[3] Among the questions asked are whether the patient can pay bills, access distant sites outside the home, and use the telephone. In this way any specific problem can be addressed and hopefully eased. Occupational therapy has a major role in assessment of these areas. However, it should be noted that overall improvement in function and the maintenance of flexibility provided by physiotherapy intervention is of great importance.

Because impairment of function has important social consequences, an assessment of *Social* issues is included in the CGA. The nature of any social problems depends very much on the individual's circumstances. It is vital to determine the usual living arrangements of the patient and the type of help available from family members at home. As the disease progresses, patients will inevitably require increasing assistance. The nature of the help depends on the available help and the type of dysfunction. Patients living alone will require help earlier on. Those with live-in helpers in the form of family members need careful monitoring to avoid strain on and ultimate burnout of the care provider. With advanced disease, institutional care is usual after the patient has reached the point of total dependency requiring 24-hour nursing care. The healthcare team has an ongoing role to play in helping patients and their families to cope with this and also to deal with the inevitable problems that affect PD patients. Ongoing assessment and treatment of problems as they arise help a great deal in enhancing the quality of life for these debilitated individuals.

Once the areas of function have been addressed, a careful assessment must be made of all the medical or *Pathophysiological Problems* of the patient. All problems interact, and the treatment of one area may well interefere with the management of another area. For this reason, each problem is identified and any associated medication noted. It requires experience, skill, and working with the patient and family to modify drug regimens. Often decisions need to be made whereby some problems cannot be optimally treated because of the development of significant side effects and the negative impact on the disease. Patients on multiple drug therapy may well have multiple side effects or a negative impact on function in various areas. By carefully listing all drugs being taken by the patient, the possible areas of modification can be identified and dosage reduction begun. This is particularly important when the patient is experiencing such side effects as cognitive impairment or postural hypotension from drugs.

MANAGEMENT OF COGNITIVE IMPAIRMENT

It is now well recognized that an increasing proportion of patients with PD develop cognitive impairment with progress of the disease. In some patients this is due to the coincident development of a dementia, such as that due to Alzheimer's disease. For others it is part of the PD process, and these patients develop a subcortical dementia. Cognitive impairment can be detected quite early on in the course of the disease,[11] and some cognitive problems, such as spatial disorientation, are not improved by drug therapy.[12] The net result is declining cognitive or intellectual function with advancing age, and this presents special management problems. These problems are usually not helped by antiparkinsonian drugs such as dopamine.[13] The most important areas of concern are with supervision of medication and the patient's ability to cooperate, understand, and continue with rehabilitation and other forms of treatment; to manage his or her own affairs and take part in decision making about personal health and future care; to operate a motor vehicle; and finally behavioral problems that impose a strain on care providers as well as increasing the risk to the patient and others.

Medication Management

An important principle in the management of any patient receiving multiple medications is to simplify the medication regimen. All interacting or potentially interacting drug combinations should be modified. There are excellent computer programs and also printed materials for help in this process. Only those drugs that enhance the quality of life or are lifesaving should be continued. Any medications with significant side effects or which depress function should be stopped. Often this will only be determined by actually stopping the medication and monitoring the patient closely. When this is done, it can be assumed that the patient will be receiving the minimal number of drugs possible. In the frail elderly patient with PD, this may well be a number of drugs, perhaps four or five, some of which will be taken three or four times a day. The patient with even mild cognitive impairment or memory failure can run into significant difficulties. In the early stages of drug and dosage reduction, dispensing aids can be provided, along with adequate education and training of the patient. For a time this may be all that is required. As the problem advances, a family member or professional may need to set up the dispensing aid. Eventually, someone will have to take over the supervision and administration of the patient's drugs. This is not always easy, and is frequently met with resistance by the patient, who may view this as an important part of independence and control of one's own destiny. However, it is important and can be achieved with careful counselling. Patients can improve significantly when their drugs are taken correctly with the right timing.

Rehabilitation

With progressive cognitive impairment, many PD patients have increasing difficulty in learning new tasks. Furthermore, many cannot follow instruction easily with regard to their body parts. The physiotherapist has to adopt a variety of strategies to overcome these difficulties. This does not mean that physiotherapy is not worth trying. Instead, many PD patients will be very much helped by regular physiotherapy. The therapist has to realize that often, particularly after a gap of a few days, the patient may well be back at the starting point, with no recollection of what was taught on the previous visit. Thus, interventions should be frequent. Sessions should be relatively short because the patient's attention span may not be long. The therapist needs to help the patient "click in" to familiar movements or patterns, and sometimes must even finesse the patient into some activity that will enhance strength or flexibility but will not be recognized as a formal exercise routine by the patient. Strategies such as dancing or marching can be incorporated. It requires a special kind of therapist, one who is happy dealing with the elderly and who is patient and compassionate yet firm and prepared, to push the patient a little. In order to accommodate these patients, physiotherapy can be accomplished in the home setting. Alternatively, in a hospital department, special sessions will need to be set up. Ideally, these patients should attend special facilities designed for their needs, Geriatric Day hospitals, or, if circumstances warrant it, GEM or Restorative Care (Geriatric Rehabilitation) Units.

Competency

Patients with PD in its advanced stages experience considerable difficulty in looking after themselves because of their physical limitations. When cognitive impairment is superimposed on this, the situation is much more difficult, and all problems and challenges are compounded. It requires familiarity and awareness of the issues to determine that the patient is cognitively impaired. A geriatric health care team must have expertise and a significant investment of time to determine when the cognitive impairment is impairing the patient's competency and the time has come for others to take over management of certain functions. The areas of concern are with ability to manage affairs, such as finances. Information will have been gathered in the CGA by collecting information on instrumental activities of daily living. A time may be reached when the patient is convinced that all is well and that he or she is doing well, but where judgement is significantly impaired and the patient can no longer cope. Careful assessment is required to determine competency and the point at which decision making must be taken over. It is important to stress that this is not something that is done lightly and that it should only be handled by those with the expertise. An important principle is that even patients who cannot balance their checkbooks and make decisions about living on their own nevertheless participate in decision making about their lives, and that it is vital to get their assent to any therapeutic intervention. Only then will cooperation be achieved and the chances of a successful outcome be improved.

Ability to Operate a Motor Vehicle

Obviously the question of operating a motor vehicle comes to the fore in patients with PD, owing to their physical limitations. However, many patients can, if optimally treated, retain their abilities. With cognitive impairment, the problems of functional capability are compounded, and this represents a very difficult area of practice. Suffice it to say that this is something of which the treatment team must be aware and must monitor. Patients early on in the course of dementia, from Alzheimer's disease or secondary to the PD itself, develop increasing difficulty with driving. They are unable to follow instructions and have difficulty in reacting appropriately in new and challenging situations.

Behavioral Problems

With cognitive impairment comes the risk of delirium. This is often precipitated by medications, as has been discussed. The patient with dementia may also have a worsening of problems from medications, and may therefore lose inhibitions and develop behavioral problems. Angry outbursts, verbal abuse, occasional physical abuse, sexual disinhibition, wandering, and endangering others by risk-taking actions in a kitchen are all problems that these patients face. The therapist must be aware of these problems and requires skill in handling these patients. It is wise to avoid direct confrontation and thus prevent outbursts. When outbursts do occur, the approach should be to try to determine the reason for them and then to gently divert the patient. Familiarity with surroundings and personnel is important. Each health professional who deals with such patients should be aware that the onset of delirium or a decline in function, which may be manifest as an inability to cooperate in rehabilitation or an inability to perform tasks of which the patient was previously capable, indicates that the frail parkinsonian patient is ill. This is referred to as a geriatric presentation and indicates the need for a careful and comprehensive evaluation, and for the management of any fresh, intercurrent problems.

CONCLUSION

It can be seen that management of patients with PD is complex. Many of these patients are old and have associated problems. In order for them to function at an optimal level, all of their problems should be addressed in an orderly and competent fashion. There is much more to the management of PD than diagnosis and drug therapy. At all stages of the illness, education of patient and family is extremely valuable. Such education rests with all members of the healthcare team: the physician, nurse, and physiotherapist, and the occupational therapist in particular. A holistic approach that pays attention to lifestyle, nutrition, regular exercise, and supportive relationships is required in all patients. The need for this approach is compelling when there are many interacting problems and when the patient can be considered frail. Much of the education can be achieved within the setting of lay organizations, such as Parkinson's societies. There is an increasingly important role for specialized geriatric services, with the availability of a full healthcare team and an array of geriatric programs in the management of these challenging patients. The disease will not be cured or eradicated; the problems will remain and in our present state of knowledge the disease will inevitably progress and the patient will get worse. But the patient and family will be able to cope more easily with the disability it brings, and a life of enhanced quality will be added to advancing years.

REFERENCES

1. The Parkinson Study Group. Effect of Deprenyl on the progression of disability in early Parkinson's disease. N Engl J Med 322(21):1526, 1990
2. Reynolds GP, Elsworth JD, Blau K et al: Deprenyl is metabolized to methamphetamine and amphetamine in man. Br J Clin Pharmacol 6:542, 1978
3. Lawton MP, Brody EM: Assessment of older people: self-maintaining and instrumental activities of daily living. Gerontologist 9:179, 1969.
4. Folstein MS, Folstein S, McHugh PR: Mini-mental state—a practical method for grading the cognitive state of patients for the clinician. J Psychiat Res 12:189, 1975.

5. Girotti F, Soliven P, Carella F, et al: Dementia and cognitive impairment in Parkinson's disease J Neurol Neurosurg Psychiatry 51:1498, 1988.

6. Golden WE, Lavender RC, Metzer WS: Acute Postoperative confusion and hallucinations in Parkinson's disease. Ann Intern Med 111:218, 1989.

7. Levin BE, Llabre MM, Weiner WJ: Parkinson's disease and depression: psychometric properties of the Beck Depression Inventory. J Neurol Neurosurg Psychiatry 51:1401, 1988.

8. Mathias S, Nayak USL, Isaacs B: Balance in the Elderly Patient: "Get-up and Go" Test. Arch Phys Med Rehab 67:387, 1986.

9. Podsiadlo D, Richardson S: The timed "Up and Go"; a test of basic functional mobility for frail elderly persons. J Am Gerontol Soc 39:142, 1991.

10. Granger CV, Albrecht GL, Hamilton BB: Outcome of comprehensive medical rehabilitation: measurment by PULSES profile and Barthel Index. Arch Phys Med Rehab 60:145, 1979.

11. Levin BE, Llabre MM, Weiner WJ: Cognitive impairments associated with early Parkinson's disease. Neurology 39:557, 1989.

12. Hovestadt A, De Jong GJ, Meerwaldt JD: Spatial disorientation in Parkinson's disease; no effect of levodopa substitution therapy. Neurology 38:1802, 1988.

13. Mohr E, Fabbrini G, Williams J, et al: Dopamine and memory function in Parkinson's disease. Mov Disord 4:113, 1989.

3 | Neural Transplantation Therapy

Alan Fine
Douglas D. Rasmusson

Parkinson's disease (PD) is a common, devastating neurodegenerative disorder for which there is currently no cure. Its pathology is largely restricted to the loss of one cell type in the central nervous system, the neurons that utilize dopamine as their neurotransmitter. Preliminary experiments on animal models of PD have suggested that impaired motor function can be greatly improved by grafting dopamine-secreting cells into appropriate sites in the brain. These results have led to initial attempts to apply the technique of neuronal grafting to human PD patients in Mexico, Sweden, China, Cuba, England, the United States, and Canada. This review discusses the rationale behind this procedure, the evidence that has led scientists to believe that it can be successfully applied to human patients, and some of the problems that still need to be resolved.

RATIONALE

Parkinson's disease is well suited to the application of neural grafts because it results from the degeneration of a discrete population of neurochemically homogeneous neurons, leaving the rest of the brain, including the normal targets of those neurons, essentially intact. The dopaminergic neurons involved have their cell bodies in the substantia nigra and send their axons into the striatum (the caudate nucleus and putamen). In PD, brain dopamine levels and the numbers of dopaminergic cells decrease progressively. However, because of various compensatory mechanisms, clinical symptoms of PD appear only when dopamine depletion exceeds 80 percent[1] and cell loss exceeds 50 percent.[2] Thus, much of the damage has been done before the patient is even diagnosed as having PD. Since the cause of the degeneration is unknown, it is at present impossible to stop this progression, which leads to ever increasing incapacitation culminating in death. Current therapies are only palliative at best. As a result of the progressive degeneration, drug treatment usually becomes less effective over time. For these reasons the replacement of dopaminergic neurons via transplantation is seen as a promising means of restoring the patient's function by replacing the lost or unhealthy cells.

Since a neural pathway from the substantia nigra to the striatum has been lost in this disease, it would seem most natural to implant new dopaminergic cells into the substantia nigra. However, to produce its effect, dopamine must be able to act on the postsynaptic cells in the striatum; unfortunately, nerve fibers have proven unable to grow over the long distances from the substantia nigra to the striatum in the adult central nervous system; such grafts of dopaminergic neurons into the substantia nigra have been ineffective in animal models of parkinsonism.[3] The direct infusion of dopaminergic agonists into the striatum, on the other hand, can ameliorate experimental parkinsonism in rats. Thus, dopamine may function, at least in part, without requiring the specific, point-to-point connections associated with the classical neuroanatomic pathways. This is in concert with findings about other "neuromodulators", such as acetylcholine and noradrenaline, which may act over a greater distance and for a longer time than are associated with the traditional synapse.

Two sources of donor tissue have already been used for clinical transplants of dopamine-secreting cells. The normal adrenal medulla synthesizes dopamine in large amounts as a precursor to adrenaline. The adrenal chromaffin cells are of neuroectodermal origin and, in the presence of glucocorticoids from the adrenal cortex, produce the enzyme phenylethanolamine-N-methyl transferase (PNMT), which converts noradrenaline to adrenaline. In the absence of glucocorticoids and in the presence of nerve growth factor, these cells will cease production of PNMT, with the result that they secrete dopamine and noradrenaline but not adrenaline.[4] Under these conditions, they can also develop axons and make synaptic connections.[4] A possible advantage of using adrenal tissue is that a patient's own adrenal medulla could be used as the donor tissue (autografts), thereby avoiding the possibility of tissue rejection.

Several problematic assumptions underlie the use of adrenal autografts. First, the plasticity of adrenal medullary cells may diminish with age[5]; since PD is generally a disease of the elderly, it is not clear that adrenal autografts from these patients would be useful. Second, it is possible that the disease process will have damaged the adrenal medullary cells as well. For example, methlyphenyltetra-hydropyridine (MPTP), a drug that produces PD in humans and other primates, affects cells of adrenal glands as well as the brain in monkeys.[6,7]

A second source of dopamine-secreting cells has been the developing human brain. From animal studies, it appears that the most successful grafts are of tissue obtained after the cells have ceased to divide but before they have begun to grow their axons. If they are taken at later stages of development, the inevitable cutting of these axons during tissue preparation may be fatal to the cells. On the other hand, if grafts are prepared from very early tissue, when cells are still actively dividing, the effect of subsequent transplant growth may resemble that of a brain tumor. Furthermore, the dopamine-secreting cells would be diluted by other, irrelevant cell types derived from the same early tissue. In the case of the dopamine-secreting cells of the human substantia nigra, the period of the 6th to the 12th weeks of gestation appears to be optimal for transplantation, since at this stage the cells are postmitotic but have only limited arborizations.[8]

A major concern with grafts made from one individual to another of the same species (allografts) is the possibility of tissue rejection. There are several reasons why the degree of kinship between donor and host may have less effect on the survival of neural transplants than had previously been expected, but the most important appears to be that the majority histocompatibility molecules that distinguish tissue from different individuals of the same species are normally absent from the surface of neurons.[9,10] The molecules that distinguish tissue from different species, however, are present on fetal neurons. Thus, grafts between members of different species (xenografts) will generally be rejected unless the immune system is suppressed by cyclosporin or other drugs. Such immunosuppression may have undesirable side effects, rendering the use of animal fetuses as donors for transplantation into humans an unfavorable alternative at the present time.

THE TRANSPLANTATION PROCEDURE

Transplantation requires the preparation of donor tissue as well as insertion of this tissue into the host. In the case of adrenal autografts, the adrenalectomy is performed at the time of transplantation. Neural tissue may be implanted either as a block of tissue or as a suspension of dissociated cells. Preparation of fetal neuronal tissue may be done immediately before transplantation; alternatively, tissue may be refrigerated or frozen (cryopreserved) for days before use. (The probability of fetal pathology in the case of spontaneous abortion would make such fetuses an unsatisfactory source of tissue for transplantation.) The technique most commonly used for induced abortion during the first trimester is suction curettage, which invariably fragments the fetus. The fragment containing the fetal midbrain, the locus of the substantia nigra precursor cells, is identified and dissected free of extraneous tissue. These cells are then dissociated and their viability assessed. Tissue from a single fetus may be sufficient for a single transplantation.

The donor is prepared with guide cannulae inserted into the appropriate region of the basal ganglia using standard stereotaxic techniques. A suspension of fetal cells is taken up into a microsyringe fitted with needles of the appropriate length and is injected stereotaxically at coordinates determined individually by prior brain scanning. Injections at several sites within the host brain allow for implantation throughout the neuronally depleted structure. Possible sources of morbidity include surgical infection, excessive growth of the graft, which could compress the forebrain regions into which it is introduced, and imbalances in mood or personality owing to inappropriate secretion of neurotransmitters.

EXPERIMENTAL EVIDENCE IN ANIMALS

The first reported attempts to transplant neural tissue in mammals were made by Thompson,[11] but his transplants of cerebral cortex from adult cats to dogs were unsuccessful. Dunn[12] was the first to demonstrate that transplanted cortex could survive for up to 3 months when taken from immature (10-day-old) rats; she also observed that surviving grafts tended to be those that were richly vascularized. These findings were confirmed by LeGros Clark,[13] who successfully transplanted cortex from rabbit embryos to 6-week-old rabbits. That the surviving neurons were in fact derived from the graft was demonstrated by using radioactively labeled thymidine, which is incorporated into DNA during its synthesis in the donor.[14]

Animal models of PD generally involve the destruction of the dopaminergic projections from the substantia nigra to the striatum. Recent studies have most often used the neurotoxin 6-hydroxydopamine (6-OHDA) to destroy dopaminergic cells and terminals on one side of the brain, leading to asymmetric movement, or rotation.[15] More recently, nonhuman primate studies have been done, using MPTP to induce a parkinsonian syndrome.[16]

The first demonstrations of functional effects of intracerebral neural grafts were done in 1979 by Perlow and collaborators[17] and by Björklund and Stenevi[18]; their findings have been repeated and extended in dozens of laboratories.[19–22] It is likely that diffuse release of dopamine from the grafts accounts for at least some of their effects, since both adrenal medullary grafts[23] and nigral grafts[17] placed in a cortical cavity above the denervated striatum or in the lateral ventricle can ameliorate impaired behaviors. Moreover, infusion of dopamine into the denervated striatum over a 2-week period reduces rotation, suggesting a reduction in supersensivity in the denervated neurons.[24] Other graft-mediated effects appear to depend on the growth of dopamine fibers into the host striatum, where they can form synapses on deafferented cells.[25,26] While most of these synapses appear normal, some are organized in dense pericellular "baskets" that appear to be unique to graft-derived inputs. Grafts also appear to receive synaptic inputs from the host brain. Bolam et al.[27] found five neurochemically distinct types of synapses on dopaminergic graft neurons, resembling normal connections from the striatum to the substantia nigra. Electrophysiologic evidence also supports the functionality of synaptic connections with grafted dopaminergic neurons; thus, for example, neurons within the graft were responsive to stimulation of other areas of the brain.[28]

Few reports have been published about functional effects of fetal neuronal transplants in monkeys.[29–32] Transplantation of fetal ventral mesencephalon into the caudate nucleus of two African Green monkeys at 3 to 4 weeks after treatment with MPTP led to rapid improvement in a subjective parkinsonian rating as early as 2 days after surgery.[29] Transplantation into other parts of the brain produced a brief, transient improvement. Similar positive results were subsequently reported by the same investigators, with a slightly larger group of 10 MPTP-treated rhesus monkeys (three with fetal grafts and the remainder as various controls).[31] Some degree of functional recovery was reported in all three graft-recipient animals, with substantial increases in the cerebrospinal fluid (CSF) levels of dopamine and L-dopa in two. Fine et al.[32] studies marmosets rendered parkinsonian by MPTP. After their symptoms had stabilized, they received either dopaminergic grafts or control grafts of non-dopaminergic tissue. The dopaminergic grafts produced a marked improvement, whereas those animals with nondopaminergic grafts showed little or no improvement after 1 to 2 months. Postmortem histologic techniques showed the dopaminergic grafts to be viable. Similar positive results have been reported by Bankiewicz et al. at the National Institutes of Health (NIH) and by Wyatt et al. at the National Institutes of Mental Health (NIMH) (personal communications). Significantly, both groups failed to detect improvements in monkeys receiving adrenal medullary autografts. The evidence to date indicates that although adrenal medullary autografts can survive in the striatum, the cells in these grafts are not as able to extend fibers or make synaptic connections with striatal neurons as are cells of the fetal substantia nigra.[33] Application of nerve growth factor to adrenal medullary grafts may be necessary to enhance fiber outgrowth.[34]

RESULTS OF NEURAL TRANSPLANTATION
IN HUMANS

The first transplantation of adrenal medullary cells into the brain of a patient with PD was done in 1982 in Sweden, and reported by Backlund et al.[35] In this first trial, medullary tissue from the patient's own adrenal gland was transplanted into the caudate nucleus. While no significant deleterious effects were observed, the motor symptoms of PD improved only briefly and to a modest degree. In a subsequent study, two patients received unilateral adrenal autografts to the putamen.[36] One of these patients, a 46-year-old man, displayed improved motor performance in the limbs contralateral to the transplantation site during the first 2 days after surgery. During the next 2 months, his periods of normal function were also longer than before transplantation. However, these improvements subsequently disappeared, and at 6 months after the surgery the patient considered his condition to be similar to what it was before the operation. The second patient, a 63-year-old man, reported minor improvement in balance and gait, lasting for about 2 months after the transplantation. Positron emission tomography (PET) showed no improvement in dopamine receptor density in the patient's putamen. The authors concluded that transplantation of adrenal tissue to the putamen had transient beneficial effects in patients with severe PD. No deleterious effects were observed in these patients over a period of 14 months.

More dramatic effects following autografts of adrenal medullary tissue were reported by Madrazo and colleagues.[37] Two young male patients (both under 40 years of age) received grafts placed in contact with one caudate nucleus adjacent to the lateral ventricle. Bilateral improvements in motor impairments were seen in both patients almost immediately after their recovery from the transplant surgery. Five months after surgery, one patient was able to walk and eat without help and "did not require drugs." Rigidity and akinesia were "practically absent on both sides" of the body, while tremor was dramatically reduced on the right (transplant) side and slightly reduced on the left side. Ten months after transplantation, this patient was playing soccer with his son. Rigidity and tremor were also abolished in the second patient. Despite the great interest aroused by this report, it presented a number of serious difficulties: the authors did not evaluate their patients by widely used, standardized methods before and after surgery; the patients were uncharacteristically young for PD; greater improvement was seen ipsilateral than contralateral to the graft; only 2 of 11 patients receiving transplants were described in the article; CSF catecholamine levels were not determined; and postmortem histologic examination in 2 patients who died failed to confirm survival of the graft.

There have now been over 200 adrenal medullary autografts for PD performed in North America; a voluntary registry of these procedures is at Emory University. Some improvement has been obtained in several centers in the United States when the operation was performed on young, less severely affected patients, but improvements have been less often obtained with those who are older and more severely affected. According to the Emory registry, at least four such patients in the United States have died from complications of the adrenalectomy.

Transplantation of fetal tissue was first described by Madrazo et al.[38] in two PD patients. The tissue was obtained from a spontaneously aborted, 13-week fetus and grafted to the caudate nucleus. The patients, a 50-year-old man with PD of 9 years duration and a 35-year-old woman with a 5-year history of PD, were evaluated using standardized procedures such as videotape, computed tomographic (CT) scan, electromyography, evoked potentials, neuropsychologic testing, and the Unified Parkinson's Disease Rating Scale (UPDRS). As a result of transplantation of fetal substantia nigra, the first patient's UPDRS score improved from 59 to 45. The second patient received a graft of fetal adrenal medullary tissue and her UPDRS score of 71 improved to 35. A crucial shortcoming of the report by Madrazo et al. was the reliance on a single rating score to characterize their patients' status, since such patients usually experience a great deal of fluctuation in their condition.

Additional successful fetal neural transplants have recently been reported by Lindvall et al.[39] A 49-year-old man received tissue from the ventral mesencephalon of four 8- to 9-week fetuses. Multiple injections of tissue were made into the putamen contralateral to the patient's most seriously affected limbs. Extensive behavioral testing was begun 11 months before the transplantation and continued throughout 5 postoperative months. The indications of improved function included a decrease in rigidity, increased speed in repetitive movements, and decreased severity during periods of disease activity. Lindvall et al. also used PET to determine that the dopaminergic neurons had survived and that indices of dopamine synthesis were improved.

ETHICAL CONSIDERATIONS

Two kinds of ethical question are commonly raised about the type of transplants described here. The first relates to the use of tissue from aborted fetuses. Might the therapeutic use of fetal tissue encourage abortion, motivate conception for the sole purpose of donating fetal tissue, and ultimately lead to the sale of fetal tissue? The second relates to the potential risk of this procedure for the PD patient.

The procurement of fetal tissue for transplantation might conceivably motivate abuse if it were the sole reason for abortion. However, the frequency of routine abortions for independent reasons already far exceeds projected needs for transplantation: each year, over 1.3 million pregnancies are voluntarily terminated in the United States alone. Approximately two-thirds of induced abortions are performed at stages appropriate for neural transplantation (i.e., between the 6th and 11th weeks of gestation). Approximately 100,000 new cases of PD are diagnosed each year in the United States, and not all of these would be satisfactory candidates for transplantation surgery. Thus, even if dopaminergic neurons could be isolated from only one in 10 currently available fetuses, the supply of fetal neural tissue from legal and independently motivated abortions substantially exceeds anticipated demand.

There have been suggestions that the use of fetal tissue may lead to an increase in the number of abortions by providing new reasons for abortion, such as for providing donor tissue for a genetically related recipient. However, as described above, no immunologic advantage appears to be gained in this way. Financial motives could also contribute to the practice of conceiving solely to provide fetal tissue if it could be sold. At present, the sale of human organs is prohibited in the United States and Canada, a prohibition that includes the sale of human fetal tissue. In general, it appears that these possible abuses can be prevented by reasonable measures, such as prohibiting the targeting of fetal tissue to any specific recipient.[40]

A second concern is whether the risk to the recipient is warranted. Human fetal neural transplantation is at present an experimental procedure, and an unsatisfactory outcome is possible. The grafts may be without effect or may even compromise brain function and exacerbate parkinsonian symptoms. However, the risks associated with the procedure must be considered in the light of the progressive and terminal course of PD. These risks may be acceptable because of the benefits of success to the patient. The decision should be the patient's, without coercion and after thorough discussion of the procedure and its forseeable risks.

EVALUATION OF THE SUCCESS OF TRANSPLANTATION

As suggested by the speed with which transplantation has been clinically applied, there is a natural human tendency to look only for positive results and to disregard the negative. Nevertheless, because there are so many unanswered questions with respect to transplantation, it is important to emphasize the criteria that should be met if this treatment is to become widely used. These criteria are as follows:

1. Behavioral assessment of the patient by a variety of objective measures and by independent observers. The need for independent observers is obvious

and essential for any study in which the experimenter's knowledge of treatment and desire for success can influence the measurements taken. The need for diverse measures is the consequence of the range of behavioral symptoms that make up PD. These symptoms vary, not only between patients but within a patient, according to time of day, activity level, time since the last dose of medication, and other factors. Clinical parameters that may be tested include resting tremor, rigidity, dexterity, standing posture, postural stability, gait, and bradykinesia. Oculomotor impairment is also often present in PD. This can be assessed along with other visual functions. Possible cognitive impairments can also be determined, using a wide range of neuropsychologic tests. Comparison of pre- and post-transplantation measures provides a much broader analysis of the effects of the graft than can be obtained from a single behavioral measure.

2. Evaluation of the survival of the graft. Much of the detailed study of whether grafts have survived and formed synapses in the host brain can only be done with histologic examination of postmortem tissue. Nevertheless, the use of PET techniques, such as by Lindvall et al.,[39] allows the imaging of functional dopaminergic structures in the patient during recovery. An alternative but more invasive technique is the measurement of metabolites of dopamine in the CSF.

3. A more difficult issue to evaluate is the extent to which any improvement in behavior results from graft-derived dopamine function as opposed to other possible effects of the transplantation surgery. Examples include the surgical disruption of the blood-brain barrier and induction of regeneration and sprouting by the patient's own dopaminergic neurons. Moreover, it has been noted[41] that lesions of the caudate nucleus that are similar to the cavities produced for transplantation have been reported to relieve tremor[42] and bradykinesia.[43]

4. Some sites within the striatum may be better than others for receiving the transplant. Based on a rapidly expanding knowledge of their function, it appears that the basal ganglia include at least five parallel but largely independent circuits, only one of which is exclusively motor in function. The others are involved in preparation for movement, eye movements, and limbic functions.[44] There is already evidence in the primate MPTP model that placement of a graft into different regions of the striatum will influence different aspects of the parkinsonian syndrome.[45] Thus, it may be that patients in whom different symptoms predominate may require transplants to different parts of the basal ganglia.

5. Identification of the conditions likely to promote graft survival and innervation. It is obviously important that the techniques involved in isolating and handling donor cells before transplantation be improved to maximize cell viability. It is not known, however, whether it would be best to separate dopaminergic from nondopaminergic cells, with transplantation only of the former, or whether the nondopaminergic cells and particularly glial cells are necessary to enhance the survival and formation of connections of dopaminergic cells with the host brain. With respect to the treatment of the donor, it is possible that inserting guide cannulae into the basal ganglia several days before transplantation may stimulate, by local trauma, the production of growth factors within the host brain and thereby facilitate recovery. The production of a small cavity

several days before transplantation improves the survival of grafted neurons in the rat,[46] owing to soluble factors released into the cavity.[47] Such growth factors may also facilitate the growth of axons and formation of new synapses by the dopaminergic neurons. The role of the target tissue in functional recovery is also indicated by Björklund and colleagues' observations[48] that when dopaminergic neurons were transplanted into the cerebral cortex and striatum, only those in the striatum (their normal target) sent out appreciable numbers of fibers, although the cells survived in both sites.

6. An important unanswered question is the long-term prognosis for patients receiving transplants, even if there is substantial improvement in the short term. It is possible, for example, that the disease process that has destroyed the patient's own dopaminergic neurons will attack and destroy the grafted neurons. However, the relatively slow progress of PD suggests that such a phenomenon, even if it occurs, would still leave the grafted cells functional for an extended period.

ROLE OF THE PHYSIOTHERAPIST

Given these many unknowns, it may appear premature to ask what part the therapist might play in the management of the parkinsonian transplant recipient. However, given the rapid progress in this area and the speed with which human clinical trials are being initiated, it seems not unlikely that transplantation patients will soon become commonplace. The most obvious immediate need is for reliable and objective assessment of their behavioral function. As mentioned earlier this should take place over many months, include a wide range of tests, and take note of flucuations with respect to drug therapy and periods of disease activity and inactivity. Assessment is necessary throughout the postsurgical period, not only shortly after transplantation, when the evidence seems to suggest that recovery is likely, but in the long term, for which there are no data as yet. After years of greatly reduced mobility, PD patients frequently experience muscular atrophy from muscle disuse. Vigorous care of the early PD patient to prevent secondary complications may well preclude the time necessary for post-transplant rehabilitation. Moreover, patients who have undergone transplantation may be faced with the arduous task of relearning simple and complex motor skills. The speed with which muscle strengthening and relearning occur will surely depend on the quality of physiotherapy. However, the type of post-transplantation therapy that might be most effective in assisting the recovery of function is largely unknown.

REFERENCES

1. Riederer P, Wuketich St: Time course of nigrostriatal degeneration in Parkinson's disease. J Neural Trans 38:277, 1976
2. McGeer PL, McGeer EG, Suzuki JS: Aging and extrapyramidal function. Arch Neurol 34:33, 1977

3. Dunnett SB, Björklund A, Schmidt RH et al: Intracerebral grafting of neuronal cell suspensions. IV. Behavioural recovery in rats with unilateral 6-OHDA lesions following implantation of nigral cell suspensions in different forebrain sites. Acta Physiol Scand (suppl)522:29, 1983
4. Unsicker K, Reiffert B, Ziegler W: Effects of cell culture conditions, nerve growth factor, dexamethasone and cyclic AMP on adrenal chromaffin cells in vitro. Adv Biochem Pharmacol 25:51, 1980
5. Tischler AS, Greene LA: Phenotypic plasticity of pheochromocytoma and normal adrenal medullary cells. Adv Biochem Pharmacol 25:61, 1980
6. Fine A, Reynolds GP, Nakijima N et al: Acute administration of 1-methyl-4-phenyl-1,2,3,6-tetrahydropyridine affects the adrenal glands as well as the brain in the marmoset. Neurosci Lett 58:123, 1985
7. Stoddard SL, Tyce GM, Ahlskog JE et al: Decreased catecholamine content in parkinsonism adrenal medullae. Exp Neurol 104:22, 1989
8. Nobin A, Björklund A: Topography of the monoamine neuron systems in the human brain as revealed in fetuses. Acta Physiol Scand (suppl)388:1, 1973
9. Lampson LA, Siegel G: Defining the mechanisms that govern immune acceptance or rejection of neural tissue. In Gash DM, Sladek JR Jr (eds): Transplantation into the mammalian CNS. Prog Brain Res 78:243, 1988
10. Widner H, Brundin P, Björklund A, Moller E: Survival and immunogenicity of dissocated allogenic fetal neural dopamine-rich grafts when implanted into the brains of adult mice. Exp Brain Res 76:187, 1989
11. Thompson WG: Successful brain grafting. NY Med J 51:701, 1890
12. Dunn EH: Primary and secondary findings in a series of attempts to transplant cerebral cortex in albino rat. J Comp Neurol 27:565, 1917
13. LeGros Clark WE: Neuronal differentiation in implanted foetal cortical tissue. J Neurol Psychiatry 3:263, 1940
14. Das GD, Altman J: Transplanted precursors of nerve cells: Their fate in the cerebellums of young rats. Science 173:637, 1971
15. Ungerstedt U: Postsynaptic supersensitivity after 6-hydroxy-dopamine induced degeneration of the nigro-striatal dopamine system. Acta Physiol Scand (suppl)367:69, 1971
16. Burns RS, Chiueh CC, Markey S et al: A primate model of Parkinson's disease: selective destruction of substantia nigra, pars compacta dopaminergic neurons by N-methyl-4-phenyl-1,2,3,6-tetrahydropyridine. Proc Natl Acad Sci USA 80:4546, 1983
17. Perlow MJ, Freed WJ, Hoffer BJ et al: Brain grafts reduce motor abnormalities produced by destruction of nigrostriatal dopamine system. Science 204:643, 1979
18. Björklund A, Stenevi U: Reconstruction of the nigrostriatal dopamine pathway by intracerebral nigral transplants. Brain Res 177:555, 1979
19. Björklune A, Stenevi U (eds): Neural Grafting in the Mammalian CNS. Elsevier, Amsterdam, 1985
20. Fine A: Transplantation in the central nervous system. Sci Am 82:52, 1986
21. Azmitia EC, Björklund A (eds): Cell and Tissue Transplantation into the Adult Brain. Ann NY Acad Sci 495, 1987
22. Björklund A, Lindvall O, Isacson O, et al: Mechanism of action of intracerebral neural implants: studies on nigral and striatal grafts to the lesioned striatum. Trends Neurosci 10: 509, 1987
23. Freed WJ, Morihisa JM, Spoor E et al: Transplanted adrenal chromaffin cells in rat brain reduce lesion-induced rotational behaviour. Nature 292:351, 1981

24. Strömberg I, Johnson S, Hoffer B, Olson L: Reinnervation of dopamine-denervated striatum by substantia nigra transplants: immunohistochemical and electrophysiologial correlates. Neuroscience 14:981, 1985
25. Freund TF, Bolam JP, Björklund A et al: Efferent synaptic connections of grafted dopaminergic neurons reinnervating the host neostriatum: a tyrosine hydroxylase immunocytochemical study. J Neurosci 5:603, 1985
26. Mahalik TJ, Finger TE, Strömberg I, Olson L: Substantia nigra transplants into denervated striatum of the rat: Ultrastructure of graft and host interconnection. J Comp Neurol 240:60, 1985
27. Bolam JP, Freund TF, Björklund A et al: Synaptic input and local output of dopaminergic neurons in grafts that functionally reinnervate the host neostriatum. Exp Brain Res 68:131, 1987
28. Arbuthnott G, Dunnett SB, McLeod N: Electrophysiological properties of single units in dopamine-rich mesencephalic transplants in rat brain. Neurosci Lett 57:205, 1985
29. Redmond DE, Sladek JR, Roth RH et al: Fetal neural grafts in monkeys given methylphenyltetrahydropyridine. Lancet 1:1125, 1986
30. Bakay RAE, Barrow DL, Fiandaca MS et al: Biochemical and behavioural correction of MPTP Parkinson-like syndrome by fetal cell transplantation. Ann NY Acad Sci 495:623, 1987
31. Sladek JR, Collier TJ, Haber SN et al: Reversal of parkinsonism by fetal nerve cell transplants in primate brain. Ann NY Acad Sci 495:641, 1987
32. Fine A, Hunt SP, Oertel WH et al: Transplantation of embryonic marmoset dopaminergic neurons to the corpus striatum of marmosets rendered parkinsonian by 1-methyl-4-phenyl-1,2,3,6-tetrahydropyridine. Prog Brain Res 78:479, 1988
33. Morihisha JM, Nakamura RK, Freed WJ et al: Transplantation techniques and the survival of adrenal medulla autografts in the primate brain. Ann NY Acad Sci 495:599, 1987
34. Strömberg I, Herrara-Marschitz M, Ungerstedt U et al: Chronic implants of chromaffin tissue into the dopamine-denervated striatum. Effects of NGF on graft survival, fiber outgrowth and rotational behavior. Exp Brain Res 60:335, 1985
35. Backlund E-O, Granber P-O, Hamberger B et al: Transplantation of adrenal medullary tissue to striatum in parkinsonism. First clinical trials. J Neurosurg 62:169, 1985
36. Lindvall O, Backlund E.-O, Farde L et al: Transplantation in Parkinson's disease: two cases of adrenal medullary grafts to the putamen. Ann Neurol 22:457, 1987
37. Madrazo I, Drucker-Colin R, Diaz V et al: Open microsurgical autograft of adrenal medulla to the right caudate nucleus in two patients with intractable Parkinson's disease. N Engl J Med 316:831, 1987
38. Madrazo I, Leon V, Torre C et al: Transplantation of fetal substantia nigra and adrenal medulla to the caudate nucleus in two patients with Parkinson's disease. N Engl J Med 318:51, 1988
39. Lindvall O, Brundin P, Widner H et al: Grafts of fetal dopamine neurons survive and improve motor function in Parkinson's disease. Science 247:574, 1990
40. Fine A: The ethics of fetal tissue transplantation. Hastings Center Report, 18:5, 1988
41. Van Manen J, Speelman JD: Caudate lesions as a surgical treatment in Parkinson's disease. Lancet 1:175, 1988
42. Myers R: Surgical experiments in the therapy of certain "extrapyramidal" disease: a current evaluation. Acta Psychiatr Neurol Scand (suppl)67:7, 1951
43. Speigel EA, Wycis HT, Szekely EG et al: Role of the caudate nucleus in parkinsonian bradykinesia. Conf Neurol 26:336, 1965

44. Alexander GE, DeLong MR, Strick PL: Parallel organization of functionally segregated circuits linking basal ganglia and cortex. Annu Rev Neurosci 9:357, 1986
45. Dunnett SB, Annett L: Nigral transplants in primate models of parkinsonism. p. 27. In Lindvall O, Björklund A, Widner H (eds): Intracerebral Transplantation in Movement Disorders. Elsevier Science Publishing, Amsterdam, 1991
46. Lewis ER, Cotman CW: Neurotransmitter characteristics of brain grafts: Striatal and septal tissues form the same laminated input to the hippocampus. Neuroscience 8:57, 1982
47. Nieto-Sampedro M, Lewis ER, Cotman CW et al: Brain injury causes a time-dependent increase in neuronotrophic activity at the lesion site. Science 217:860, 1982
48. Björklund A, Stenevi U, Schmidt RH et al: Intracerebral grafting of neuronal cell suspensions. II. Survival and growth of nigral cells implanted in different brain sites. Acta Physiol Scand (suppl)522:11, 1983

4 | Motor Control in Parkinson's Disease

George E. Stelmach
James G. Phillips

An understanding of the structures and processes involved in the control of movement can better assist in the detection, diagnosis, and assessment of motor dysfunction.[1-3] This chapter is concerned with disturbances of motor control caused by Parkinson's disease (PD) and what this disorder of movement can reveal about the role of the basal ganglia in the normal control of movement. A consideration of the motor functions that PD has impaired or spared can in turn provide starting points for the physical therapy of patients with the disease.[4]

Parkinson's disease affects motor control in several ways:

1. Some motor functions are lost or impaired. Patients are bradykinetic, having problems performing fast movements.
2. There may be some disinhibition of some functions. Patients show tremor at rest, and their limbs are rigid, resisting passive stretching.
3. Compensation may occur through the use of intact functions. Patients show an increased reliance on visual feedback.

FUNCTIONAL LOSS

Parkinson's disease affects several neurotransmitter systems.[5,6] In particular, the degeneration of one dopaminergic system, the nigrostriatal tract, is pronounced. The impact of dopamine replacement therapy on patients' movements demonstrates that the dopaminergic nigro-striatal system has a key role in the control of movement.[7] Treatment with L-dopa (a dopamine precursor) or dopamine agonists (e.g., bromocriptine) dramatically improves patients' control of movement.[8] The functional loss caused by PD is of interest to researchers, since the identification of functional loss may provide insights into the role of the basal ganglia in the control of movement.[9]

This chapter focuses initially on the symptoms of akinesia and bradykinesia in PD.[6,10] Patients with PD have in some fashion lost the ability to produce fast, smooth movements. They show reductions in spontaneous and associated movement, are slow in initiating movements (akinesia), and are slow and halting during the execution of their movements. They also fatigue easily (bradykinesia). Both their akinesia and bradykinesia are debilitating symptoms.[10]

The symptoms of PD can fluctuate during chronic therapy,[11] and the motor functions of patients with the disease show a greater variation than that of any cognitive functions (e.g., ref. 12). Indeed the motor disturbances of PD may tend to limit the expression and assessment of cognitive functions.[13]

To appreciate the functional losses caused by PD, it is necessary to consider the processes involved in the normal control of movement. In normal subjects, movements can be prepared in advance and then run off ballistically from a program (open-loop control).[14] In this case, the required preparation can be inferred from the response latency.[15] Movements can also be controlled and guided during their execution by using feedback (closed-loop control),[14] in which case the amount of guidance can to some extent be inferred from the duration of the movement.[16] While movements that are prepared in advance tend to be rapid and smooth, with symmetric phases of acceleration and deceleration, feedback-guided movements are typically slower, jerkier, and asymmetric in their acceleration and deceleration phases.[17,18]

By comparison, patients with PD clearly have problems using predictive information to prepare their movements,[19] and it has been suggested that the disease causes problems in the programmed control of movements.[9] A consideration of the preparatory processes of patients with PD may throw some light on the functional losses causing akinesia in these patients.

AKINESIA

It is thought that akinesia in PD is the result of impaired preparatory processes.[9] Researchers examine preparatory processes by measuring patients' reaction times (RTs). This is a cognitivist approach that assumes that action involves a series of preparatory computations that can be inferred from delays in responding.[20] In the measurement of reaction time, patients are asked to initiate their movements quickly in response to a stimulus. The time between stimulus presentation and response initiation (reaction time, or RT) is used as an index of movement preparation; the greater the RT, the greater the preparation required for the movement. By systematically varying the complexity of movements (e.g., movement length or direction) during an experiment, researchers can assess the time taken to prepare specific movement parameters.[21,22] Investigators using RT-based techniques are interested in disproportionate increases in patients' RTs in movements that increase in difficulty along a specific dimension. Cognitivist approaches assume that PD patients will show disproportionate slowness in tasks that require functions that are lost or impaired.

Despite this expected slowness, studies reporting deficits in patients with PD typically report a different pattern of results.[21,23] Rather than the increased RT expected from the performance of normal control subjects as a baseline, PD patients show little increase in RT with increasing task difficulty. Thus, for example, although slow in initiating movements with a single stimulus-reponse alternative (simple RT), PD patients are not much slower than normals when initiating movements with two stimulus-response alternatives (choice RT).[23]

Many studies that have compared simple and choice RTs have found that PD patients have impaired simple RTs[24–26]; see also ref. 27). Unfortunately, the specific functional loss underlying this effect is difficult to discern on the basis of comparisons of simple and choice RTs, since the two measures confound the number of stimuli and responses.[28] We will thus focus on systematic studies of the preparatory processes of patients with PD which reveal that they are less likely than normals to use preparatory cues.

While normal subjects are quick to initiate their responses when a warning signal has been provided, PD patients do not benefit from a warning signal.[24,29] Studies using informative warning signals (precues) have shown that PD patients are slow in responding and do not seem to make as much use of the precue as normals,[30,31,32,33] because incorrect precues tend not to inconvenience them. They seem to perceive but do not act on the basis of advance information.

This is better illustrated in studies of the preparation of movement sequences. Patients with PD are less likely to prepare a sequence of movements in advance than are normal individuals. While RT is normally related to sequence length, Stelmach and colleagues[34] found that PD patients' RTs did not increase with the number of finger taps in a response sequence. Stelmach and co-workers[23] also found that PD patients were able to prepare finger taps in advance when there was a straightforward relationship between stimulus and response, but not when the stimulus–response relationship was more complicated. Similarly, Harrington and Haaland,[35] in examining the initiation of sequences of repetitive and heterogeneous hand postures, found that PD patients could prepare sequences of repetitive movements but were less likely to prepare a sequence of alternating movements. It would seem that patients with PD cannot prepare complicated or novel movements.[23,36]

PD patients have problems performing tasks that require more attention (novel or complicated tasks), but it is not clear whether they have reduced attentional resources (primary functional loss) or simply require more of their attention to plan their movements (secondary functional compensation). Parkinson[37] himself observed that even simple movements require considerable concentration in these patients.

PD patients have problems performing tasks that require more attention (novel or complicated tasks), but it is not clear whether they have reduced attentional resources (primary functional loss) or simply require more of their attention to plan their movements (secondary functional compensation). Parkinson[37] himself observed that even simple movements require considerable concentration in these patients.

Attentional processes in PD have been examined using dual task paradigms. These procedures assume that the attentional resources of PD patients are limited, and infer the attentional requirements of a primary task from the additional delays that the task causes in the performance of a concurrent secondary task.[38] While normal subjects show decrements in performance in comparisons of their single- and dual-task performance, patients with PD are very slow during their performance of a single task and show little further impairment during dual task performance.[29,39] This suggests that they are always performing as if they have little available spare attentional capacity.[40]

Which functions are impaired by PD? There has been discussion about the extent to which the functional losses seen in patients with PD are the product of a single functional deficit[40] as opposed to a number of separate deficits.[40,42] For example, Brown and Marsden[40] have considered whether PD patients have a generalized attentional deficit, while Hallett[42] has reasoned that the akinesia and bradykinesia in PD are the products of two distinct functional impairments.

It is not clear how a generalized attentional impairment could cause the observed deficits in PD patients' movements. Goldenberg[43] suggested that if PD patients have a general attentional deficit, they should show disproportionate problems when nonmotor tasks are examined using dual-task procedures. In fact Goldenberg,[43] did not find a general attentional deficit when PD patients performed verbal and visuospatial memory tasks. Such data suggest that PD patients have a specific impairment that is yet to be identified.

The observed deficits in PD patients' motor control suggest that they have some problem of response selection or initiation that makes their movements laborious rather than smooth and effortless. This suggests that they have problems in disengaging their attention from movement and performing their movements automatically. Possibly these problems in the initiation of movement lead to the bradykinesia seen in PD patients. In this case, bradykinesia would be considered a compensation for deficits in preparatory processes.

BRADYKINESIA

The bradykinesia observed in PD could be the product of impaired preparatory processes. When movements are not prepared in advance, they can be controlled during their execution through feedback guidance.[16] An increase in the duration of a specific movement suggests that the movement requires more feedback guidance. In addition to moving in a slow, jerky manner, patients with PD show an increased reliance on visual feedback.[19,44] While normally rapid ballistic movements are typically smooth, with symmetric acceleration and deceleration phases,[17,18] PD patients show the jerky, asymmetric acceleration–deceleration profiles[45,46] normally expected of visually guided movements.[18] While it might seem possible that the bradykinesia in PD is a secondary effect of akinesia, Hallett[42] has argued that this may not be the case. Rather Hallett[42] has suggested that the akinesia and bradykinesia in PD are the products of different physiologic mechanisms. Bradykinesia is more consistently observed than akinesia in PD,[47] and the degree of bradykinesia does not correlate with the degree of akinesia in these patients.[47,48] In particular, dopamine improves the bradykinesia but not the akinesia in the disease, as measured by simple RT,[25,29] suggesting that the akinesia and bradykinesia involve different mechanisms.

Hallett and Khoshbin[49] have suggested that PD patients are bradykinetic because they have difficulty in energizing their muscles. They observed that as compared with normal subjects, patients with the disease require more cycles of agonist and antagonist muscle activity to produce a movement. They hypothesized that the patients' initial agonist muscle activity is insufficient and that the patients need to employ more small bursts of activity to produce the same movement as normal subjects, requiring a greater number of bursts of muscle activity to produce faster or longer movements.

It is unlikely that PD patients' failure to appropriately energize their muscles is a result of reduced muscle strength, even though Koller and Kase[50] have reported decreased muscle strength in isometric tasks in these patients. Research has found that bradykinesia is not simply the result of problems in energizing muscles.[44,51,52] For example, Yanagawa et al.[52] used electrical stimulation to demonstrate that reductions in muscle force are not a product of impairments in the peripheral neuromuscular system. Tetanic stimulation produced normal levels of force output in patients with PD. Bradykinesia would seem to be the result of problems within the central nervous system.

Studies such as that of Yanagisawa et al.[53] have suggested that PD patients have problems not with the amounts of force they can produce, but in producing forces rapidly. Indeed, there are consistent reports that patients with PD are slower and more variable in their movements.[44,51,54,55] Unfortunately, the mechanisms involved are not yet clear. It seems that when patients produce movement forces accurately,[56,57] their force production is slow and jerky. Conversely, when patients produce movement forces at near normal speeds, their force production is highly variable.[55]

Patients with PD can be slow and accurate or faster and inaccurate in their movements, trading speed for accuracy. However, they have a reduced capacity to control their movements; they are always slower or less accurate than normal subjects. While there is also a relationship between speed and accuracy in normal subjects, PD patients are abnormal in that their movements become far more variable and inaccurate when they move at faster speeds.[55] Montgomery and Nuessen[54] have suggested that as compared with that of normal subjects, the speed/accuracy function in PD patients has a poorer slope and intercept.

Various investigators have suggested that PD patients cannot scale their movement forces appropriately, such that their movements fall short of any target.[44,51,54,55] We have seen that the speed and accuracy of their performance varies. It now seems that the slowness of PD patients may be a function of task constraints and accuracy requirements.[41,58] They are more likely to demonstrate deficits in novel tasks with precise accuracy requirements.[41,59] Indeed, in tasks with precise accuracy requirements, it is possible to find situations in which PD patients actually produce too much rather than insufficient force. This can be seen in a study by Muller and Abbs[60] of precision grip in PD patients, in which they were required to grip an object without dropping it (this requires forces greater than the weight of the object). Although PD patients are typically thought to produce insufficient force, the patients in this study overgripped, producing more force than was required to grip the object.

Data suggest that patients with Parkinson's disease have a reduced capacity to control the speed and accuracy of movement forces, and that this is exacerbated in novel or precision tasks. Given that PD patients show a slowness and uncertainty in their movements, it is perhaps necessary to consider whether their akinesia and bradykinesia are conservative motor-control strategies brought on by the disinhibition of other functions.[4]

DISINHIBITION

Research in the motor behavior of PD patients has been primarily directed toward the identification of functional losses producing akinesia and bradykinesia. It may, however, be important to distinguish the effects of akinesia and bradykinesia in PD from positive symptoms such as rigidity and tremor. We will discuss the extent to which rigidity and tremor may contribute to PD patients' slowness in initiating and executing movements. We suggest that it is unlikely that rigidity or tremor are the sole determinants of the observed slowness and jerkiness in these patients' movements, since parkinsonian symptoms occur somewhat independently.[48] It is, for example, possible to find patients with intense rigidity but only moderate bradykinesia.[10]

Rigidity

The mechanisms producing parkinsonian rigidity are unclear,[59] but it seems that spinal or long-latency reflexes are disinhibited.[10] Patients with PD demonstrate increased muscle activity at rest, abnormal amounts of activity in long-latency reflexes,[61] and abnormalities in the reciprocal innervation of muscles.[62]

It has been suggested that rigidity may prevent PD patients from performing fast, smooth movements. For example, Ohye et al.[63] suggested that rigidity and bradykinesia in PD were due to antagonistic muscle co-contraction. However, it is unlikely that rigidity causes the bradykinesia seen in the disease, since there is evidence that bradykinesia is independent of rigidity. For instance, Caligiuri[64] found no relationship between rigidity and speed of orofacial movements in PD patients. Yanagawa and colleagues[52] have similarly demonstrated no relationship between the rigidity and speed of limb movements.

Tremor

Parkinsonian tremor occurs at rest at a frequency of 4 to 5 Hz. It is thought to arise from a disinhibition of pacemaker cells in the thalamus.[65]

Freund[66] has suggested that tremor limits the speed with which PD patients can control their movements. Unless they move below a certain speed (e.g., 2 to 4 Hz), their tremor entrains their movements,[67,68] such that control is lost as their movements hasten,[68,69] and that their movements occur at a characteristic frequency associated with their tremor.

Tremor is unlikely to be the sole cause of the jerkiness and hesitancy in PD patients' movements. Clinically, parkinsonian tremor occurs at rest,[10] and it is possible to select patients with minimal tremor. Phillips et al.[70] have observed jerkiness and hesitancy in the movements of PD patients with minimal tremor. The jerkiness of the patients' movements was not regular and did not occur at frequencies associated with tremor (5 to 8 Hz), suggesting that bradykinesia was not simply a function of tremor.

To better understand basal ganglia function in PD, we have considered the functional losses caused by the disease and considered whether these losses can be explained by disinhibition of other functions. To better define functional loss we will now consider which functions are maintained.

COMPENSATION

Because research in PD has tended to focus on the identification of specific functional losses caused by the disease,[9] the sparing of function has been of less direct interest for understanding the function of basal ganglia. The consideration of those functions that are intact indirectly assists in understanding the function of the basal ganglia by ruling out some of its potential roles in the control of movement. On the other hand, the sparing of function is perhaps of direct relevance for physical therapy in PD. In healthy individuals, a number of processes that appear to be spared by PD contribute to the control of movement.[14,15] In overview, it appears that yet unidentified impairments in the programming and execution of movements cause PD patients to rely on the visual guidance of movements.

Accurate movements require an appreciation of distance and direction. Patients with PD appear to have a normal perception of distance.[23,71,72] Indeed, studies reporting perceptual deficits in PD patients appear to have been confounded by motor deficits, lack of appropriate age-matched controls,[73] or both. It has been suggested that fast movements are controlled by generalized motor program that is supplied with parameters to meet the demands of specific motor tasks.[74] It would appear that this general program is intact in PD patients, since their movements retain the overall shapes of the same movements in normals,[75] but are reduced in scope. An elegant experiment by Stelmach et al.[34] showed that the specification of movement parameters, such as direction, arm versus leg movement, and extent of movement, is normal in PD patients. While there appears to be some problem in the activation or energization of their movements, various studies have shown that PD patients can use visually or verbally presented feedback to control their movements.[44,56,57,76] They can be trained to vary the length and duration of their movements,[76] and can be trained to vary the amounts for force they produce isometrically or isotonically.[44,56] They also appear to move more slowly to improve the accuracy of their movements by processing visual feedback.[19,59] The intact functions would seem to assist in compensating for PD patient's functional impairments.

The programs and processes specifying and modifying movement parameters are intact in PD patients, but they appear to be overloaded. Perhaps the mechanisms that disengage effort from movement are damaged.[40] Their movements may be uncertain because the correct motor impulse has not been clearly selected from its alternatives.

To what extent, then, can PD patients compensate and regain some of their lost fluency of movement? They would seem to be able to learn new skills, but require more practice than normals to accomplish this. For example, while PD patients exhibit a characteristically longer simple RT, Worringham and Stelmach[77] found that their simple RT improves with practice. They can to some extent learn to preprogram their movements. There are, however, signs that the learning process is abnormal. Unlike normal subjects, PD patients do not show the signs of "warming-up" during the acquisition of a skill.[78] Whle normal subjects show a rapid improvement at the beginning of a training session (perhaps because they access and tune a motor program), patients with PD perform poorly, and show only gradual improvement during a training session. Such data again suggest that PD patients have difficulty in accessing a motor program.

BASAL GANGLIA FUNCTION

The locations of the basal ganglia, and the wealth of pathways surounding them, have made them difficult to study through the use of electrical stimulation or lesioning.[79] Marsden[9] suggested that an understanding of the specific functional losses caused by PD can provide insight into the role of the basal ganglia in the control of movement.

Various functions have been ascribed to the basal ganglia. Some researchers have suggested that they have several roles.[42,80,81] Marsden[79] has suggested that the basal ganglia play a role in the automatic execution of movement. From the evidence reviewed, it does seem that they assist in the disengagement of attention from ongoing movement.[40] It has also been suggested that the basal ganglia serve as a gate or channel that selects movements.[79] In PD this gate is open, while in Huntington's disease this gate is shut.[79,82] The basal ganglia seem to have an energizing role, activating a specific movement after it has been chosen by other, presumably cortical mechanisms.

The study of movement disorders provides insight into the role of brain structures in the control of movement, potentially providing converging evidence about the mechanisms involved in movement control. This chapter illustrates some of the emerging isomorphism between neurophysiologic and cognitive psychological accounts of motor control, outlining brain structures involved in the control of movement, and their functions. In turn, the assessment of function is the basis of rehabilitation. As functional loss is identified, PD no longer seems immutable.[4]

While PD may impair the disengagement of attention from movement and may affect the activation of movements, it leaves other motor functions intact. Patients with PD can, for example, prepare their movements[34] and control the length and duration[44,76] of their movements when given feedback. Recent observations that patients with PD can benefit from practice[77] show that physical therapy may have a role in helping these patients.

REFERENCES

1. Hallett M: Analysis of abnormal voluntary and involuntary movements with surface electromyography. Adv Neurol 39:907, 1983
2. Martin, WRW, Calne DB: Imaging techniques and movement disorders. p. 4–16. In Marsden CD, Fahn S (eds): Movement Disorders. Butterworths, London
3. Yanagisawa N: EMG characteristics of involuntary movements. p. 142. In Bruyn SW, Roos RAC, Buruma OJS (eds): Dyskinesias. Actua Sandoz, Vol. 7. Sandoz, Uden, Switzerland, 1984
4. Grimm RJ, Nashner LM: Long-loop dynscontrol. p. 70. In Desmedt JE (ed): Cerebral Motor Control in Man: Long Loop Mechanisms Karger, Basel, 1978
5. Fahn S: The medical treatment of movement disorders. p. 249. In Crossman AR, Sambrook MA (eds): Neural mechanisms in disorders of movement. John Libbey, London, 1989
6. Jankovic J: Pathophysiology and clinical assessment of motor symptoms in Parkinson's disease. p. 99. In Koller WC (ed): Handbook of Parkinson's Disease. Marcel Dekker, New York, 1987
7. Newman RP, Calne DB: Parkinsonism: Physiology and pharmacology. p. 39. In Shah NS, Donald AG (eds): Movement Disorders. Plenum Medical Book Company, New York, 1986
8. Lieberman AN, Goldstein M: Parkinson's disease: Current concepts. p. 83. In Shah NS, Donald AG (eds): Movement Disorders Plenum, New York, 1986
9. Marsden CD: The mysterious motor function of the basal ganglia: The Robert Wartenberg Lecture. Neurology 32:514, 1982
10. Delwaide PJ, Gonce M: Pathophysiology of Parkinson's signs. p. 59. In Jankovic J, Tolosa E (eds): Parkinson's disease and movement disorders. Urban & Schwarzenberg, Baltimore, Munich, 1988
11. Obeso JA, Grandas F, Vaamonde J et al: Motor complications associated with chronic levodopa therapy in Parkinson's disease. Neurology 39, (suppl 2): 11, 1989
12. Girotti F, Carella F, Grassi MP: Motor and cognitive performances of parkinsonian patients in the on and off phases of the disease. J Neurol Neurosurg Psychiatry 49:657, 1986
13. Korczyn AD, Inzelberg R, Treves T et al: Dementia of Parkinson's disease. p. 399. In Yahr MD, Bergmann KJ (eds): Advances in Neurology. Vol. 45. Raven Press, New York, 1986
14. Stelmach GE: Motor control and motor learning: the closed-loop perspective. p. 93. In Kelso JAS (ed): Human motor Behavior: An Introduction. Lawrence Erlbaum Associates, Hillsdale, New Jersey, 1982
15. Stelmach GE: Information-processing framework for understanding human motor behavior. p. 63. In Kelso JAS (ed): Human Motor Behavior: An Introduction. Lawrence Erlbaum Associates, Hillsdale, New Jersey, 1982

16. Howarth CI, Beggs WDA: The control of simple movements by multisensory information. p. 125. In Heuer H, Kleinbeck U, Schmidt K-H (eds): Motor Behaviour: Programming, Control, and Acquisition. Springer-Verlag, Berlin, 1985

17. Hogan N, Flash T: Moving gracefully: quantitative theories of motor coordination. Trends Neurosci 10:170, 1987

18. Nagasaki H: Asymmetric velocity and acceleration profiles of human arm movements. Exp Brain Res 74:319, 1989

19. Flowers KA: Visual "closed-loop" and "open-loop" characteristics of voluntary movement in patients with Parkinsonism and intention tremor. Brain 99:269, 1976

20. Stelmach GE, Hughes BG. Cognitivism and future theories of action: Some basic issues. p. 3. In Prinz W, Sanders AF (eds): Cognition and Motor Processes. Springer-Verlag, Berlin, 1984

21. Stelmach GE, Worringham CJ, Strand EA: The programming and execution of movement sequences in Parkinson's disease. Int J Neurosci 36:55, 1987

22. Wing AM, Miller E: Basal ganglia lesions and the psychological analyses of the control of voluntary movement. p. 242. In Ciba Foundation Symposium 107: Functions of the Basal Ganglia. Pitman, London, 1984

23. Stelmach GE, Phillips JG, Chau AW: Visuo-spatial processing in parkinsonians patients. Neuropsychologia 27:485, 1989

24. Bloxham CA, Mindel TA, Frith CD: Initiation and execution of predictable and unpredictable movements in Parkinson's disease. Brain 107:371, 1984

25. Pullman SL, Watts RL, Juncos JL, Sanes JN: Movement amplitude choice reaction time performance in Parkinson's disease may be independent of dopaminergic status. J Neurol Neurosurg Psychiatry 53:279, 1988

26. Sheridan MR, Flowers KA, Hurrell J: Programming and execution of movements in Parkinson's disease. Brain 110:1247, 1987

27. Brown VJ, Robbins TW: Simple and choice reaction time performance following unilateral striatal dopamine depletion in the rat. Brain 114:513, 1991

28. Zelaznik H: Precueing response factors in choice reaction time—word of caution. J Motor Behav 10:77, 1978

29. Bloxham CA, Dick DJ, Moore M: Reaction times and attention in Parkinson's disease. J Neurol Neurosurg Psychiatry 50:1178, 1987

30. Sharpe MH: Distractibility in early Parkinson's disease. Cortex 26:239, 1990

31. Sharpe MH: Patients with early Parkinson's disease are not impaired on spatial orienting or attention. Cortex 26:515, 1990

32. Wright MH, Burns RJ, Geffen GM, Geffen LB: Covert orientation of visual attention in Parkinson's disease: An impairment in the maintenance of attention. Neuropsychologia 28:151, 1990

33. Yamada T, Izyuuinn M, Schulzer M, Hirayama K: Covert orienting attention in Parkinson's disease. J Neurol Neurosurg Psychiatry 53:593, 1990

34. Stelmach GE, Worringham CJ, Strand EA: Movement preparation in Parkinson's disease: the use of advanced information. Brain 109:1179, 1986

35. Harrington DL, Haaland KY: Sequencing in Parkinson's disease. Brain 114:99, 1991

36. Day BL, Dick JPR, Marsden CD: Patients with Parkinson's disease can employ a predictive strategy. J Neurol Neurosurg Psychiatry 47:1299, 1984

37. Parkinson J: An Essay of the Shaking Palsy. Sherwood, Neely, and Jones, London, 1817

38. Glencross DJ: Control and capacity in the study of skill. p. 2. In Glencross DJ (ed): Psychology and Sport. McGraw-Hill, Sydney, 1978

39. Goodrich S, Henderson L, Kennard C: On the existence of an attention-demanding

process peculiar to simple reaction time: Converging evidence from Parkinson's disease. Cognitive Neuropsychol 6:309, 1989

40. Brown RG, Marsden CD: Dual task performance and processing resources in normal subjects and patients with Parkinson's disease. Brain 114:215, 1991

41. Connor NP, Abbs JH: Task-dependent variations in Parkinsonian motor impairments. Brain 114:321, 1991

42. Hallett M: Clinical neurophysiology of akinesia. Revue Neurologie (Paris) 146:585, 1990

43. Goldenberg G: Performance of concurrent non-motor tasks in Parkinson's disease. J Neurology 237:191, 1990

44. Teasdale N, Phillips J, Stelmach GE: Temporal movement control in patients with Parkinson's disease. J Neurol Neurosurg Psychiatry 53:862, 1990

45. Muller F, Stelmach GE: Scaling problems in Parkinson's disease. p. 161. In Requin J, Stelmach GE (eds): Tutorials in Motor Neuroscience. Elsevier, Amsterdam, 1991

46. Wing AM: A comparison of the rate of pinch grip force increases and decreases in Parkinsonian bradykinesia. Neuropsychologia 26:479, 1989

47. Evarts EV, Teravainen H, Calne DB: Reaction time in Parkinson's disease. Brain 104:167, 1981

48. Zetusky WJ, Jankovic J, Pirozzollo FJ: The heterogeneity of Parkinson's disease: clinical and prognostic implications. Neurology 35:522, 1985

49. Hallett M, Khoshbin S: A physiological mechanism of bradykinesia. Brain 103:301, 1980

50. Koller W, Kase S: Muscle strength testing in Parkinson's disease. Eur Neurol 25:130, 1986

51. Berardelli A, Dick JPR, Rothwell JC et al: Scaling of the size of the first agonist EMG burst during rapid wrist movements in patients with Parkinson's disease. J Neurol Neurosurg Psychiatry 49:1273, 1986

52. Yanagawa S, Shindo M, Yanagisawa N: Muscular weakness in Parkinson's disease. p. 259. In Streifler MB, Korczyn AD, Melamed E, Youdim MBH (eds): Parkinson's Disease: Anatomy, Pathology, and Therapy. Raven Press, New York, 1990

53. Yanagisawa N, Fujimoto S, Tamaru F: Bradykinesia in Parkinson's disease: Disorders of onset and execution of fast movement. Eur Neurol 29, suppl. 1:19, 1989

54. Montgomery EB, Nuessen J: The movement speed/accuracy operator in Parkinson's disease. Neurology 40:269, 1990

55. Wierzbicka MM, Wiegner AW, Logigian EL, Young RR: Abnormal most-rapid isometric contractions in patients with Parkinson's disease. J Neurol Neurosurg Psychiatry 54:210, 1991

56. Stelmach GE, Teasdale N, Phillips J, Worringham CJ: Force production characteristics in Parkinson's disease. Exp Brain Res 76:165, 1989

57. Stelmach GE, Worringham CJ: The preparation and production of isometric force in Parkinson's disease. Neuropsychologia 26:93, 1988

58. Teasdale N, Stelmach GE: Movement disorders: The importance of the movement context. J Motor Behav 20:186, 1988

59. Sheridan MR, Flowers KA: Movement variability and bradykinesia in Parkinson's disease. Brain 113: 1149, 1990

60. Muller F, Abbs JH: Precision grip in Parkinsonian patients. p. 191. In Streifler MB, Korczyn AD, Melamed E, Youdim MBH (eds): Parkinson's Disease: Anatomy, Pathology, and Therapy. Raven Press, New York 1990

61. Lee RG: Pathophysiology of rigidity and akinesia in Parkinson's disease. Eur Neurol 29, suppl 1:13, 1989

62. Hayashi A, Kagamihara Y, Nakajima Y et al: Disorder in reciprocal innervation upon initiation of voluntary movement in patients with Parkinson's disease. Exp Brain Res 70:437, 1988

63. Ohye C, Tsukahara N, Narabayashi H: Rigidity and disturbance of reciprocal innervation. Confin Neurol 26:24, 1965

64. Caligiuri MP: Labial kinematics during speech with patients with Parkinsonian rigidity. Brain 110:1033, 1987

65. Findley LJ, Gresty MA: Tremor and rhythmical involuntary movements in Parkinson's disease. p. 295. In Findley LJ, Capildeo R (eds): Movement Disorders: Tremors. Oxford University Press, New York; 1984

66. Freund H-J Motor dysfunctions in Parkinson's disease and premotor lesions. Eur Neurol 29, suppl. 1, 33, 1989

67. Frischer M: Voluntary vs autonomous control of repetitive finger tapping in a patient with Parkinson's disease. Neuropsychologia 27:1261, 1989

68. Nagasaki H, Nakamura R: Rhythm formation and its disturbances—A study based upon periodic response of a motor output system. J Hum Ergol 11:127, 1982

69. Nakamura R, Nagasaki H, Narabayashi H: Disturbances of rhythm formation in patients with Parkinson's disease: Part I. Characteristics of tapping response to the periodic signals. Percept Motor Skills 46:63, 1978

70. Phillips JG, Stelmach G, Teasdale N: What can indices of handwriting quality tell us about Parkinsonian handwriting? Hum Movement Sci 10:301, 1991

71. Brown RG, Marsden CD: Visuospatial function in Parkinson's disease. Brain 109:987, 1986

72. Della Sala SD, Lorenzo GD, Giordano A, Spinnler H: Is there a specific visuospatial impairment in Parkinsonians? J Neurol Neurosurg Psychiatry 49:1258, 1986

73. Bodis-Wollner I, Marz, MS, Mitra S et al: Visual dysfunction in Parkinson's disease. Brain 110: 1675, 1987

74. Schmidt RA: The schema concept. p. 219. Ink Kelso JAS (ed): Human Motor Behavior: An Introduction. Lawrence Erlbaum Associates, Hillsdale, New Jersey 1982

75. Margolin DI: The neuropsychology of writing and spelling: Semantic, phonological, motor, and perceptual processes. Q J Exp Psychol 36A:459, 1984

76. Phillips J, Stelmach G, Teasdale N: Preliminary assessment of spatio-temporal control of handwriting in Parkinsonians. p. 317. In Plamondon R, Suen CY, Simner ML (eds): Computer Recognition and Human Production of Handwriting (pp. 317–331). World Scientific Publishing Co, Singapore 1989

77. Worringham CH, Stelmach GE: Practice effects on the preprogramming of discrete movements in Parkinson's disease. J Neurology Neurosurg Psychiatry 53:702, 1990

78. Frith CD, Bloxham CA, Carpenter KN: Impairments in the learning and performance of a new manual skill in patients with Parkinson's disease. J Neurol Neurosurg Psychiatry 49:661, 1986

79. Marsden CD: Defects of movement in Parkinson's disease. In Delwaide PJ, Agnoli A (eds): Clinical Neurophysiology in Parkinsonism. Elsevier, Amsterdam, 1985, pp 107–115

80. Brown RG, Marsden CD: Cognitive function in Parkinson's disease: From description to theory. Trends Neurosci 13:21, 1990

81. Connor NP, Abbs JH: Sensorimotor contributions of the basal ganglia: Recent advances. p. 112. In Rothstein JM (ed): Movement Science. American Physical Therapy Association, Alexandria, VA 1991

82. Stelmach GE, Phillips JG: Movement disorders: Limb movements and the basal ganglia. Phys Ther 71:60, 1990

5 | The Kinematics of Gait

James C. Wall
George I. Turnbull

The gait pattern of persons with Parkinson's Disease (PD) has been widely documented, mostly from a descriptive viewpoint. The actual gait pattern will vary with the stage of the disease. Asymmetry characterizes the early stages, but later the "typical" PD gait pattern begins to emerge. In the later pattern, the affected individual demonstrates diminishing arm swing and an overall attitude of flexion when walking,[1] with the head projecting abnormally anteriorly and the thoracic spine becoming kyphotic. The arms and legs assume a flexed and adducted posture and the patient takes increasingly shorter steps. Also evident are retropulsion and propulsion, in which PD patients take increasingly shorter but faster steps as if attempting to "catch-up" with their displaced centre of mass. The feet eventually fail to clear the surface, giving rise to the shuffling gait pattern. Freezing, in which the patient appears to be "stuck" to the floor, may occur.[2] Inept attempts to initiate a step and unsteadiness and the potential for falling become evident.[3] This gait pattern will become more pronounced as the disease progresses or as medication loses its effectiveness. One of the major manifestations of PD is the characteristic shuffling gait pattern with little or no associated movements in the upper limbs and trunk.[4]

In this chapter the kinematics of gait in PD are discussed. The discussion is restricted to descriptions of the movement pattern (kinematics) and does not detail the forces causing those movements (kinetics). We have taken this approach in an attempt to make the chapter more meaningful to the practicing clinician who has to assess PD patients with limited equipment, that is, without the force platforms and electromyographic data collection systems required for a comprehensive gait analysis. We wish to concentrate on objective measurements that can be used in the clinic to better classify Parkinsonian patients, to determine the extent of their gait deviations, and to use this information to make decisions about treatment strategies. Consequently the objective measurements herein discussed focus on the temporal and distance parameters of gait. Apart from helping to define the gait pattern of the PD patient, these measurements are also useful in monitoring the patient to determine the efficacy of the treatment being provided.

INFLUENCE OF WALKING SPEED ON OTHER PARAMETERS OF GAIT

Perhaps the single most important measurement of gait is walking speed, since virtually all other measures vary with it. In looking at Parkinsonian patients, one of the most noticeable features of their gait is the slow speed at which they walk. In healthy individuals, be they young or elderly, the gait pattern changes as walking speed decreases. Stride length decreases and stride time increases, the percentage of the stride spent in double support and total support both increase, whereas the percentage of the stride spent in single support and swing decrease.[5,6] These effects must be taken into account when attempting to determine which deviations in the PD patient's gait are due to the underlying neurologic deficit and which are due simply to the patient's very slow walking speed.

Several papers report studies of the temporal/distance gait kinematics of the PD patient. In only one of these studies did the PD patients walk at more than one self-selected walking speed with measurements made before and after the administration of levorotatory dihydroxy phenylalanine (L-dopa).[7] Since the effects of L-dopa and walking speed are the focus of this chapter we have used primarily the data from this paper for comparison with the normative data. Blin et al.[7] studied the gait patterns of six women PD patients between 61 and 85 years of age (mean 69 years). Four of the women were at Stage III of the Hoehn and Yahr scale; the remaining two were grade IV. The patients were tested in the morning before taking their medication and were again measured one hour after taking 200 mg of L-dopa. At each session measurements were made at patient-selected medium and fast walking speeds.

The normative data are taken from a group of 10 healthy young women. These women were asked to traverse an instrumented walkway[8] at five self-selected walking speeds: very slow, slow, medium, fast, and very fast. Each subject made two traverses of the walkway at each of these speeds. The mean data for each speed were then calculated.

Let us first consider walking speed. Figure 5-1 shows the range of walking speeds for the young adults together with that extracted from the study by Blin et al.[7] for PD patients before and after L-dopa administration. The range for the young adults was from 0.88 m/s to 1.74 m/s. In the Blin[7] study the subjects, before taking L-dopa, had a normal walking speed of 0.36 ($\pm$ 0.13) m/s and a fast walking speed of 0.66 ($\pm$ 0.22) m/s. After taking L-dopa these speeds increased to 0.60 ($\pm$ 0.15) and 0.92 ($\pm$ 0.28) m/s respectively, which still do not exceed the values obtained for the slow walking speed of the healthy individuals (Figure 5-1). The mean of the 21 PD patients in the study by Knutsson[4] was 0.56 ($\pm$ 10.21) m/s with a range from 0.05 to 0.94 m/s.

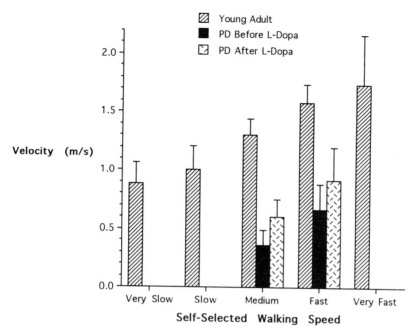

Fig. 5-1. The range of walking speeds for a group of healthy young adult females together with the data for a group of six PD patients taken from Blin et al.[7]

Stride Length

As can be seen from Figure 5-2, stride length increases with walking speed in the group of healthy individuals. The data for the PD patients also show that with an increase in walking speed, stride length increases, both before and after administration of L-dopa, but the values are below what might be predicted from the normative data. (Care must be taken when extrapolating the normative data outside of the actual range of walking speeds over which the data were collected. However, given that the speeds of the PD patients were close to the very slow walking speeds of the young adult group, this problem may not be of great significance in this instance.) Thus the data indicate that the L-dopa achieved an increase in speed along with an increase in stride length, but the stride length was still well below that of a normal subject walking at the same slow speed. Thus the L-dopa effected a speeded-up, abnormal gait pattern.

Stride Time

Figure 5-3 shows that in a group of healthy young adults, stride time decreases with increasing walking speed. This relationship is also true for the PD patients before and after L-dopa, although the values for stride time are well below those expected from the normative data. This agrees with the reduced

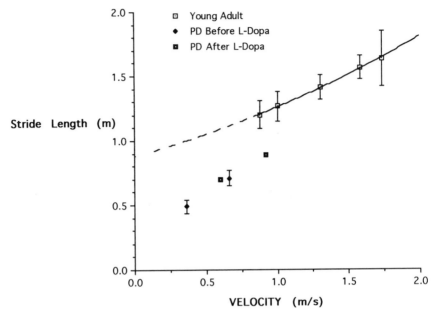

Fig. 5-2. Stride length plotted against walking speed for a group of healthy young adult females and a group of six PD patients taken from Blin et al.[7]

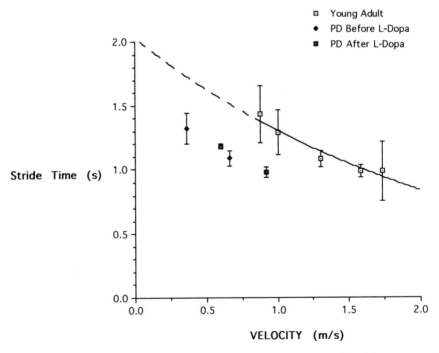

Fig. 5-3. Stride time plotted against walking speed for a group of healthy young adult females and a group of six PD patients taken from Blin et al.[7]

stride lengths shown in Figure 5-2. If a PD patient walks at the same slow speed as a normal subject and has a reduced stride length, the stride time must also be reduced because velocity is calculated by dividing distance by time. If the stride length were reduced but the stride time remained unaltered, then the velocity would be reduced because one would be covering a shorter distance in the same time. The PD patient manages to maintain the same velocity as the normal subject (who has a longer stride length) by taking more steps in a given time (i.e., an increased cadence or stride frequency). Thus the data for stride time and stride length reflect the mincing or festinating gait pattern commonly associated with PD patients.

Knutsson[4] obtained a stride time of 1.36 (± 0.29) s with a range of 0.60 to 2.5 s and a stride length of 0.75 (± 0.28) m with a range of 0.13 to 1.36 m. The patients in this study had a mean walking speed of 0.56 m/s. In a more comprehensive study (in terms of the number of subjects) Blin et al. report stride time and stride length as 1.29s (± 0.16s) and 0.57m (± 0.26m) respectively for a group of 21 PD patients walking at a velocity of 0.44m/s (± 0.20m/s).[9] These figures agree with the data in Figures 5-2 and 5-3.

Durations of Support

In Figure 5-4, the durations of the double-support phase are plotted. The normative data show the linear relationship between the duration of this, the most stable phase in the gait cycle, and walking velocity. As the velocity decreases a proportionately longer time is spent with both feet in contact with the ground. In this study, the PD patients spend far longer in the double-support phase than would be predicted from the normal data. Although actual durations cannot be determined from the data provided, the time spent in the single support phase would be reduced. This exactly parallels the findings for a group of subjects with idiopathic gait disorder of the elderly (IGDE).[10]

After taking L-dopa the patient spends less time in double support, partly as a consequence of walking at a faster speed but also because there is a slight trend towards a less abnormal pattern, although no statistics are provided to determine whether this is significant. The gait pattern is one in which the patient spends longer time in the relatively stable phase of the cycle and less when supporting body weight on one limb. This is typical of the gait pattern of people that have a fear of falling,[10] a pattern strikingly similar to that shown by PD patients. Indeed, during the study on the elderly fallers one of the subjects was diagnosed as having early PD and, as a result, had to be dropped from the study. The point here is that although the temporal and distance parameters can help to classify a PD patient, they are not definitive.

There are a number of implications from the results of these studies for clinicians involved in the care of patients with PD. The first of these relates to gait assessment, or more particularly, the objective measurement of gait.

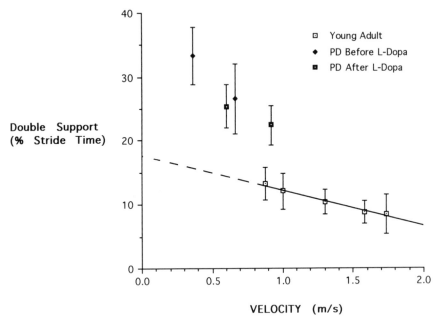

Fig. 5-4. Duration of the double-support phase, expressed as a percentage of stride time, plotted against walking speed for a group of healthy young adult females and a group of six PD patients taken from Blin et al.[7]

CLINICAL GAIT ASSESSMENT

By far the most common method of gait assessment used in the clinic is a purely subjective one,[11,12] which often results in a single comment entered in the patient's notes[13] and which is prone to misinterpretation and inaccuracy.[14] Observational gait assessment has also been found to be an unreliable clinical skill.[15-17]

The use of the videocassette recorder as an adjunct to visual inspection in the clinical gait assessment procedure has been discussed by Turnbull and Wall.[18] The recorded gait may be viewed over and over without patient fatigue. The stop action and slow motion features, common to most videorecorders, could allow the clinician to detect gait anomalies that might otherwise be missed. The recording also provides a record that allows the clinician to more easily compare a patient's gait with a normal pattern, or with that of another patient, or indeed for the same patient over the course of treatment. Kinsman[19] provides a protocol for the video assessment of the PD patient that looks at a broad spectrum of abilities such as writing and rising from a chair. The section on posture and walking has the patient start by rising from a chair without assistance from the hands to assess "start hesitation." The patient then stands upright and still for five seconds as a test of posture. When directed to do so the patient then walks 20 ft., turns unassisted, and returns to the chair. The gait is then scored primarily with reference to stride length, from 0, in which the patient "steps out well with 18–30 in stride and turns effortlessly," to 3, which is characterized by "onset of shuffling gait, steps less than 3 in. Occasional stuttering type or blocking gait. Walks on toes; turns very slowly."

In addition to aiding visual assessment, the videocassette recorder can be used to make objective measurements of gait. The protocol discussed by Kinsman[19] suggests that a walking index can be calculated by multiplying the number of steps by the time taken to stand, walk a fixed distance, and sit down. This measure does provide an objective measure in that it results in a number, but it is difficult to interpret because it incorporates a number of activities that may not be equally affected. To measure independently the time taken for each of the activities would be preferable. This protocol could be further improved by incorporating some of the gait parameters discussed above. These can be obtained in the clinic, in real time or from a videorecording, relatively simply and without requiring a great deal of time.

For example, Wall et al.[10] suggest that several of these parameters can be determined by means of a stopwatch and a marked and measured distance over which the patient must walk. Work with PD patients suggests that this distance be between 5 and 10 m. Using the stopwatch, the clinician measures the time taken (t [secs]) to cover the set distance (d [m]) and then calculates the velocity (v = d/t [m/s]). This should be done at self-selected walking speeds of slow, medium, and fast to determine the range of speeds of which the subject is capable.

The stopwatch can also be used to determine stride time. This can be done by timing a set number of strides, with a stride defined as the time taken for one complete gait cycle, usually measured from heel strike to the next heel strike by the same foot.[14] Dividing this time (T [secs]) by the number of strides (n) taken will result in stride time. One can also calculate stride length by multiplying stride time by velocity. These measurements can then be compared with the results given in this paper to help identify gait abnormalities. However, the measurements obtained in this way are the mean values for a series of strides and as such will mask the stride-to-stride variability that seems to be an important feature of the PD gait pattern.[9] If a video is being made of the patient for subsequent analysis, it is strongly suggested that the floor is marked with reference lines a known distance apart, say 5 cm, or better still a 5-cm grid, as discussed below. This would allow for measurement of individual steps and strides and consequently for the determination of variability within a walk.

A recent study tested the validity and inter-rater and intra-rater reliability of a videotape estimation method versus the ink footprint method, as described by Boenig,[20] in the measurement of step length and step width.[21] No significant differences were found between the two techniques used, indicating that the videotape method of measuring step length and step width is reliable and valid. Making these measurements requires a reference grid drawn on the floor or surface over which the subject walks. In the study by Gaudet et al.,[21] a 5-cm square grid was used. The subjects, with bright markers attached to their heels, were filmed from behind. The videotape was then advanced and stopped when the heel made contact with the ground. The X and Y coordinates of heel position were then read from the grid. This process was repeated for the next heel strike by the contralateral foot. The separation of the positions of the two heels in the direction of the walk gave step length, and the separation at right angles to this gave step width. The second step length was obtained by determining the position of the next ipsilateral heel contact. Both step lengths must be determined to measure stride length. It should not be assumed that the two step lengths will be the same, even though PD gait is regarded as symmetrical in the later stages.

A recent innovation in videocassette recorders has further increased their potential for use in the clinical assessment of gait. Videocassette recorders are available that convert the video signal into a digital format, allowing for better picture stability in slow motion and freeze-frame modes. The temporal components of the gait cycle, as seen in the data presented above, are of relatively short duration and so do not lend themselves to direct measurement with a stopwatch. This is particularly true of the double-support phases. It has even been suggested that these temporal components cannot be measured using videography given their short duration and the relatively slow video scan rate of 30 frames per second (30/s).[22] However, each of the two fields that make up a frame can be identified using the newer digital recording systems and a time code generator. This doubles the effective scan frequency to 60/s, allowing the resolution to be increased to ± 0.017 s. The validity of this technique has been determined for normal subjects walking at five self-selected walking speeds from very slow to very fast.[10] It was found that stride time and velocity could be determined reliably but that a systematic error existed in measurements of the durations of the various phases of the gait cycle. This is being investigated further to see if the error can be eliminated or explained. If the durations of the temporal phases can be so measured, it would make the videorecorder an even more powerful tool for the assessment of the patient with PD because it would allow for the determination of the double- and single-support phases that are affected in this condition. Concurrently, the videotape could be used to evaluate other parts of performance such as arm swing and posture.

MEASUREMENT OF INITIATION OF GAIT IN PD

Traditional gait analysis examines a steady pattern of walking and does not address the initiation and cessation of walking. In fact some systems include features that eliminate the gait parameters that occur at the beginning and the end of the walk to reduce the effect on data collection of acceleration and deceleration. In many PD patients, once gait has been commenced the pattern can be relatively uneventful, particularly in the earlier stages of the disease or when the patient is effectively medicated. In PD, this method of measurement tends not to accurately portray reality. It is known that PD patients suffer from disorders of movement initiation and cessation; thus, examining the features of gait pattern that only constitute the steady state, though useful, can miss features of the pattern that may be of considerable interest to the physical therapist because of their impact on functional independence. To overcome this problem, a device has been built that examines the initiation of gait in PD patients.[23] A valuable feature of this device is that it can be used to assess the effectiveness of various therapies, including rehabilitation techniques.

The device is derived from the automatic, computerized walkway system originally developed by Wall et al.[24] and later modified by Crouse et al.[8] It consists of a mat made up of a series of resistive grids driven by a stabilized, voltage-controlled current source. Metal tape attached to the sole of the patient's shoes acts to complete a current path to ground, when the foot is in contact with the mat, through the otherwise electrically isolated rods. A linear voltage-position relationship is established in which the voltage is measured at the output of the current source and the position alternates between the most proximal and distal part of the foot in contact with the walkway. The mat has independent right and left sides, which monitor data from each foot. The mat is placed at the beginning of the existing walkway, and the subject assumes a quiet standing position on this mat before walking. An operator triggers a computer that randomly determines a time period (from 0–10 s), at which time the patient receives a sound signal to commence walking. Data concerning the temporal and spatial characteristics of the initial part of the gait pattern as well as the time taken to initiate the gait cycle is thus generated. Provision has been made so that all contact points on this first mat are recorded. This feature provides data representing such characteristics of the festinating gait pattern as freezing, stutter steps, and shuffles.

To date, preliminary trials of this equipment have shown alterations in the time taken to initiate the gait cycle, possibly caused by defects of the feedforward function of the basal ganglia.[25] In addition, the first few steps have shown abnormalities in both the temporal and spatial characteristics of the gait cycle: short steps, an increased cadence, frequent errors such as scuffs, repeated steps with the same foot, and foot/floor contact discrepancies (e.g., when the patient has difficulty placing the heels on the floor). These features are well known and have been observed subjectively in the past, but this system permits more objective measurement, an important feature when attempting to evaluate performance. In terms of conservative intervention, the use of this system makes it possible to assess more accurately the role of therapeutic exercise—both preventive, in the early stages of the disease, and restorative, as the condition advances.

EFFECT OF L-DOPA ON GAIT OF PATIENTS WITH PD

In the early stages of PD, the motor manifestations are controlled by the administration of L-dopa. However, as the disease progresses, the relief obtained becomes less predictable and walking becomes affected. The gait profile of the patient during this stage is unpredictable; there is considerable variability between patients at similar stages of the disease and in the same patient from hour to hour and day to day. Typical manifestations are the appearance of the on-off syndrome, which is characterized by shifts between normal motor ability (on) and full blown Parkinson's symptoms (off). The shift can occur rapidly and randomly or may be gradual and follow a somewhat predictable course.[26] The appearance of drug-induced dyskinesias can also complicate the patient's gait pattern. Similarly, for some patients the medication will produce little improvement in PD symptoms, while for others the drug's effect will "wear off" before the next batch of medication is due to be taken. The end-of-dose deterioration, which characterizes the wearing-off effect, becomes more pronounced as drug usage increases.[27] It remains unclear whether low plasma levels of L-dopa account for the wearing-off effect but it is believed that this effect occurs when L-dopa levels drop below 50 percent. It has also been proposed that wearing-off results from an inability of the remaining dopaminergic cells to buffer changing L-dopa levels around the time of drug ingestion.[28] An increasing frequency of medication ingestion is often attempted to ensure functional benefit.[27] Regardless of the cause of this wearing-off effect, functional deterioration of motor performance is a result. Included in this is a deteriorating gait pattern towards that typically associated with PD.

Boudreau et al.[29] attempted to study this phenomenon by examining the kinematic gait parameters of 11 PD patients. These patients had reported to the same attending neurologist that increasing disability made them aware of a wearing-off of the medication before the next dose was due. The findings of this study demonstrated the difficulties encountered when attempting to study this phenomenon. The sample was composed of five women and six men between 46 and 78 years of age (Mean = 65.7 years). The time since PD onset was 3 to 34 years (mean = 11.3 years). Subjects demonstrated similar levels of impairment as a result of PD as assessed on the Webster Scale, and all were required to be able to walk at least 10 m when at their lowest level of functioning. All subjects were taking L-dopa, but the quantities varied as did the amounts of concomitant medication, such as bromocriptine. Gait kinematics were measured using the automatic, computerized walkway system described earlier. Data were collected as the subject walked at a self-selected, free speed at five-minute intervals commencing 30 minutes before routine L-dopa ingestion (around lunch time), with the final walk occurring 40 minutes after medication. Although a number of parameters such as stride time and stride length were measured along with the duration of each component of the gait pattern, only walking velocity will be discussed at this time because of its effect on these other parameters.

Gait velocity was measured in statures/s. This unit of velocity, referred to as relative speed, was proposed by Grieve and Gear[5] as a measure that accounted for differences in walking velocity as a result of height. Velocity is divided by stature and is expressed as the number of times body height is covered in overground walking in 1 s. Figure 5-5 shows the mean values and the standard deviations over the course of the data collection period. The remarkable thing about this finding is the variability found in this group of subjects. Although there is no overall evidence of a wearing-off effect, the

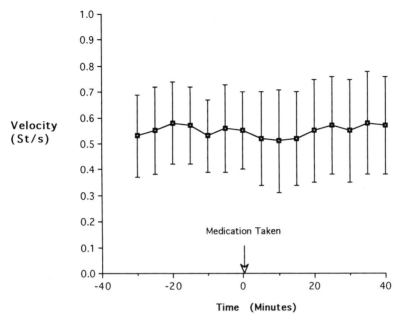

Fig. 5-5. Velocity, measured as statures/s, before and after ingestion of L-dopa.

variability between subjects was highly significant ($p = 0.0001$ when subjected to analysis of variance). It could be argued that this variability was due to the range of ages of the subjects, the variability in the time since initial onset of symptoms, and the difference in medication protocols—and these points are acknowledged. However, when it is considered that all subjects were at an equivalent stage of the disease in terms of disability levels and all had reported to the same attending physician that a wearing-off effect was occurring, the differences between subjects was less pronounced than one would at first assume. These factors are some of the reasons that render the study of people with PD difficult and highly complex. This is partly because the symptoms of PD are highly individualized. To make this point, Figure 5-6 shows the same data as the previous figure but also with the individual data from four subjects, included in the study, superimposed. This further punctuates the level of variability found and demonstrates that great caution must be exerted when drawing conclusions from the results shown in Figure 5-5.

Figure 5-7 shows two of those subjects who clearly demonstrate a wearing-off effect in their gait patterns. In particular, the data for subject 1 is extremely dramatic, ranging from a relative speed of 0.78 st/s 20 minutes before L-dopa ingestion, a speed that can be considered normal, to a low of 0.23 st/s, 10 minutes after ingestion, which is well below the slowest walking speed of a healthy person. Following this low reading, there was a rapid and dramatic alleviation of symptoms, which was associated with an increase in walking speed. In the range of slow walking speeds, subject 4 clearly derived benefit

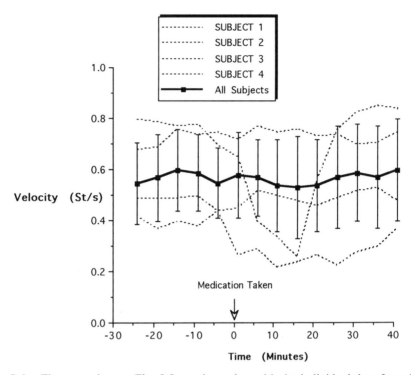

Fig. 5-6. The same data as Fig. 5-5 are shown but with the individual data from four subjects, included in the study, superimposed. This clearly demonstrates the variability found.

from the medication, but the improvement took longer to manifest than that of subject 1.

Figure 5-8 shows the data for the other two subjects, who demonstrate no evidence of a wearing-off effect as far as this gait parameter is concerned. Subject 3 walks at a very respectable speed while subject 2 walks slower than normal. However, the characteristics seen here are quite different from those of the subjects who demonstrated the wearing-off effect. It is possible that these two subjects (2 and 3) were able to adjust the way they walked to accommodate for any subjective perception of the wearing-off of the medications. However, this is not apparent from these data.

A very similar picture to that presented by the walking speed data was found in all other parameters of gait measured in this study. Significant variability in the gait between subjects, therefore, appears to be the principal finding.

The characteristics of the data obtained from subject 1 were found to be sufficiently intriguing to warrant closer inspection. Her gait pattern had been measured before the study just described, and both analyses were strikingly similar. The first time she had been tested, she had been videotaped, so it was decided to score the videotape subjectively to see if there was any relationship

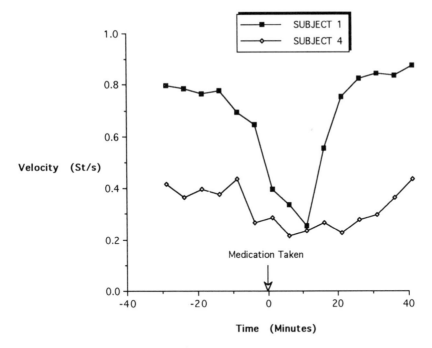

Fig. 5-7. Gait velocities of two subjects who clearly show a wearing-off effect.

between the objective gait data and the videoscore. The first time we encountered this subject, it had been decided to measure her gait kinematics every 10 minutes. However, during data collection, it was found that events were occurring quicker than had been anticipated and so this was changed to a frequency of every 5 minutes, at the 10-minute post-medication interval. This is the reason for the inconsistency in the intervals between walks during data collection. Figure 5-9 shows her relative walking speed before and after medication. Figure 5-10 shows the video assessment obtained from scoring the videotapes using the following system:

Knees Flexed	(scored as 0, absent; 1, slight; 2, marked)
Hips Flexed	(scored as 0, absent; 1, slight; 2, marked)
Thoracic Kyphosis	(scored as 0, absent; 1, slight; 2, marked)
Head Projection	(scored as 0, absent; 1, slight; 2, marked)
Arm Swing	(scored as 0, present; 1, reduced; 2, absent)
Scuffs	(number noted)
Walking	(scored as 0, steps out well; 1, steps limited slightly; 2, steps limited greatly; 3, shuffle)

Comparison of the two systems of measurement shows that the video score was highest (worst) 10 minutes after ingestion of the medication and lowest (best) 20 minutes after taking the medication. These findings are reflected in the

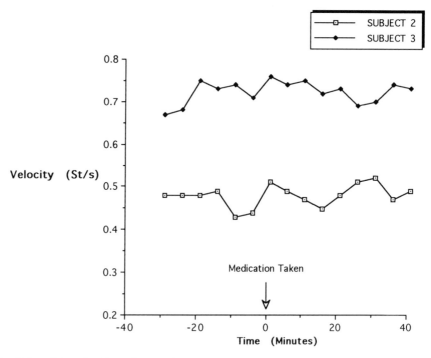

Fig. 5-8.   Gait velocities of two subjects who show no evidence of a wearing-off effect as far as this gait parameter is concerned.

data for walking speed. Similarly, the videoscore mirrors the gait measures at the other intervals. It would appear, therefore, that scoring a videotape of a patient's walk is a useful method of assessing the performance of the patient and should prove useful clinically. The advantage of the videotape is that the same walk can be viewed a number of times, thus enhancing the accuracy of the visual assessment. It is not easy to carry out this assessment technique without video because of the number of items being scored, and it is unreasonable to expect the patient to walk repeatedly while an assessment is being completed. In addition, repeated walks by the patient are likely to become altered as a result of fatigue, thus rendering the procedure invalid.

In the later stages of PD, therefore, L-dopa can have unpredictable results on the walking pattern of patients. This fact complicates physical therapy, as does the inter-subject variability. As a result, assessment and planning of treatment becomes difficult to establish on a rational basis. However, the teaching of traditional physical therapy strategies to tide the patient over until the next dose of medication takes effect is well worth considering. Similarly, the variability in the way the medication affects the patients underlines the need for comprehensive and thorough assessment and the implementation of an individualized program to suit the particular needs of a given patient.

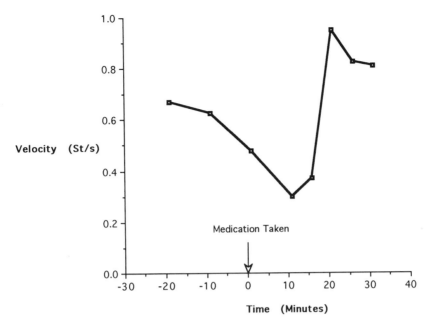

Fig. 5-9. The relative walking speed before and after medication of the subject who demonstrated dramatic wearing-off effect.

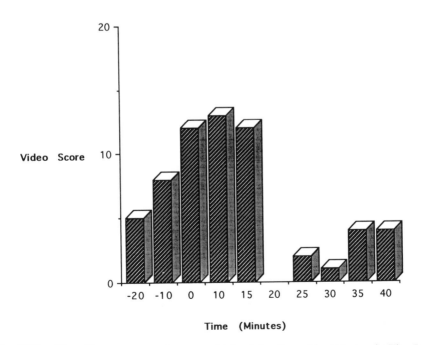

Fig. 5-10. The video assessment scores obtained for the subject shown in Fig. 5-8.

EFFECT OF VISUAL CUES ON GAIT OF PD PATIENTS

It has been known for some time that visual cues appear to improve the gait of PD patients when they are placed in front of the patient so that they can be stepped over.[30,31] Martin[32] proposed that obstacles two to three inches high produced the greatest benefit, but that brightly coloured lines were also effective. It is thought that these visual cues have a positive effect on the ability of the subject to initiate and control stepping[3,33] and may enhance the deficient motor planning process.[34] Dunne et al.[35] have also reported the effective use of an inverted walking stick as a visual cue. Bagley et al.[36] investigated the effects of visual cues on the gait kinematics of 10 PD subjects (eight men and two women) with a mean age of 77.8 years (range 69–88 years), all exhibiting mild to moderate gait dysfunction and all affected by PD to a similar extent according to the Webster evaluation. In addition to measuring relative speed as described earlier, relative stride length was measured and was defined as the proportion of body height that was covered in overground walking during one stride. The timing of the data collection was standardized to control the effects of medications.

The temporal and spatial kinematics of gait were measured, again using the automatic, computerized walkway system, first without and then with visual cues. The visual cues, yellow, triangular tubes made from light bristol board, were placed along the walkway at a customized distance for each subject. A further walk was measured to establish the presence of any carryover effect once the cues were removed.

The study concluded that there were statistically significant changes in relative stride length and step length between walks with visual cues and in the non-cued walk that immediately followed. Significant improvements were also found in stride time and in the durations of the single- and double-support phases of the gait cycle when the cue was introduced, but these significant changes did not carry over into the final non-cued walk. There was no change in walking speed between trials; thus it was concluded that the changes in the gait parameters could be regarded as a shift towards a more normal gait pattern. For example, when considering the durations of the support phases of the gait cycle (Figure 5-11), double-support time decreased significantly with the introduction of the cues with a corresponding increase in single-support time (swing on the contralateral leg). This resembles more closely a normal gait pattern in which the subject would be expected to spend approximately 60 percent of the gait cycle in support and 40 percent in swing. The cued walk approximates these rough percentages. However, the walk that followed the cued walk did not preserve this improvement.

The results of this study support the effectiveness of the introduction of visual cues as a way to improve the gait pattern of patients with PD. It is, however, unclear as to how long any carryover effect would persist. Perhaps frequent repetition of this more normal pattern would result in the preservation of these improvements once the cues were removed. In addition, the visual cues appeared to have a more pronounced effect on the spatial gait parameters

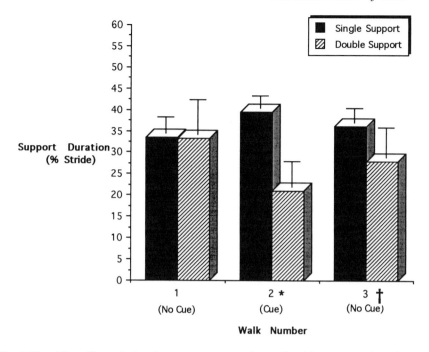

Fig. 5-11. The effect of visual cues on support times. Double-support time decreased significantly with the introduction of the cues with a corresponding increase in single-support time (swing time in the contralateral limb). However, this did not carry over into the non-cued walk that followed. (*, significantly different from walk 1; †, significantly different from walk 2.) (Modified from Bagley et al.,[36] with permission.)

than the temporal. This is probably a result of the nature of this type of cue. It would be interesting to see if time-related cues, such as auditory cues, would affect more significantly the temporal gait parameters.

CONCLUSION

Much is known, in a descriptive sense, of the gait pattern of people suffering from PD. An attempt has been made in this chapter to discuss this clinical phenomenon in the light of what is normal. The introduction of L-dopa has improved the functional abilities of these patients but has also created major difficulties for those who have tried to establish the characteristics of a typical PD gait performance. The gait of the person with PD is not as simple as it first appears, and the researching of pertinent questions is complex and fraught with the interference of confounding variables. This makes the generation of definitive answers extremely difficult.

From a clinical perspective, attempts have been made to suggest pragmatic methods to generate objective information concerning the gait pattern of this patient population. The use of emerging video technology appears to show much promise in this regard. It is only by collecting objective information to compliment subjective systems that new, improved methods of management of this disease will be developed. In addition, this becomes of paramount importance in determining the effectiveness of physical therapy in its broadest sense. It is only through close involvement by physical therapists that relevant questions will be asked and appropriate conclusions drawn. This is particularly true of gait, a functional competency of significant importance.

REFERENCES

1. Murray MP, Peterson RM: Weight distribution and weight-shifting activity during normal standing posture. Phys Ther 7:741, 1973
2. Duvoisin R: Clinical Symposia: Parkinsonism. CIBA Pharmaceutical Company, Summit, NJ, 1976
3. Franklyn S: An introduction to physiotherapy for Parkinson's disease. Physiotherapy 72:379, 1986
4. Knutsson E: An analysis of Parkinsonian gait. Brain 95:475, 1972
5. Grieve DW, Gear RJ: Relationships between length of stride step, frequency, time of swing and speed of walking for children and adults. Ergonomics 9:379, 1966
6. O'Brien M, Power K, Sanford S, Smith K, Wall JC: Temporal gait patterns in healthy young and elderly females. Physiotherapy Canada 35:323, 1983
7. Blin O, Ferrandez AM, Pailhous J, Serratrice G: Une novelle méthode d'analyse quantitative de la marche du Parkinsonien: illustration sur 6 patients. Revue Neurologique 146:48, 1990
8. Crouse JG, Wall JC, Marble AE: Measurement of the temporal and spatial parameters of gait using a microcomputer based system. Biomed Eng 9:64, 1987
9. Blin O, Ferrandez AM, Serratrice G: Quantitative analysis of gait in Parkinson patients: increased variability of stride length. J Neurol Sci 98:91, 1990
10. Wall JC, Hogan DB, Turnbull GI, Fox RA: The kinematics of idiopathic gait disorder of the elderly: A comparison with healthy young and elderly females. Scand J Rehabil Med 23:159, 1991
11. Grieve DW: The assessment of gait. Physiotherapy 55:452, 1969
12. Stanic U, Bajd T, Valencic V, Kljajic M, Acimovic R: Standardization of kinematic gait measurements and automatic pathological gait pattern diagnostics. Scand J Rehabil Med 9:95, 1977
13. Patla AE, Proctor J, Morson B: Observations on aspects of visual gait assessment: A questionnaire study. Physiotherapy Canada 39:311, 1988
14. Wall JC, Charteris J, Turnbull GI: Two steps equals one stride equals what? The applicability of normal gait nomenclature to abnormal walking patterns. Clin Biomechanics 2:119, 1987
15. Goodkin R, Diller L: Reliability among physical therapists in diagnosis and treatment of gait deviations in hemiplegics. Percept Mot Skills 37:727, 1973
16. Krebs D, Edelstein JE, Fishman S: Reliability of observational kinematic gait analysis. Phys Ther 65:1027, 1985
17. Smidt GL: Methods of studying gait. Phys Ther 54:13, 1974
18. Turnbull GI, Wall JC: The development of a system for the clinical assessment of gait following stroke. Physiotherapy 71:294, 1985
19. Kinsman R: Video assessment of the Parkinson patient. Physiotherapy 72:386, 1986

20. Boenig D: Evaluation of a clinical method of gait analysis. Phys Ther 57:792, 1977
21. Gaudet G, Goodman R, Landry M, Russell G, Wall JC: Measurement of step length and step width: A comparison of videotape and direct measurements. Physiotherapy Canada 42:12–15, 1990
22. Stuberg WA, Colerick VL, Blanke DJ, Bruce W: Comparison of a clinical gait analysis method using videography and temporal distance measures with 16 mm cinematography. Phys Ther 68:1221, 1988
23. Turnbull GI, Wall JC, Cavanagh I, Pierre P, Crouse JG: The development of an objective system to measure the initiation of gait in patients with Parkinson's Disease. Int J Rehabil Res 12:215, 1989
24. Wall JC, Dhanendran M, Klenerman L: Method of measuring temporal/distance factors of gait. J Biomed Eng 11:409, 1976
25. Rogers MW, Chan CWY: Motor planning is impaired in Parkinson's disease. Brain Res 438:271, 1988
26. Yahr MD: Movement disorders. In Rowland LD (ed): Merritt's Textbook of Neurology. Lea and Febiger, Philadelphia, 1984
27. Shaw KM, Lees AJ, Stern GM: The impact of treatment with levodopa on Parkinson's disease. Q J Med 195:283, 1980
28. Fabbrini G, Mouradian MM, Juncos JL et al: Central pathophysiological mechanisms, part 1. Ann Neurol 24:366, 1988
29. Boudreau L, O'Flaherty R, Roy L, Stewart S, Turnbull GI: The effects of L-dopa on Parkinsonian gait. Unpublished study, Halifax, Nova Scotia, 1990
30. Van Wilzelben HD: Methods of Treatment in Post Encephalitic Parkinson's. Green and Stratten, New York, 1942
31. Brenner HJ: Therapeutic Exercise for the Treatment of the Neurologically Disabled. Charles C Thomas, Springfield, MA, 1957
32. Martin JP: Locomotion and the basal ganglia. In Martin JP (ed) The Basal Ganglia and Posture. JP Lippincott, Philadelphia, 1967
33. Melnick ME: Basal ganglia disorders. Metabolic, hereditary and genetic disorders in adults. In Umphred DA (ed): Neurological Rehabilitation, 2nd Ed. CV Mosby, St Louis, 1990
34. Chan CWY: Could Parkinsonian akinesia be attributable to a disturbance in the motor preparatory process? Brain Res 386:183, 1986
35. Dunne JW, Hankey GJ, Edis RH: Parkinsonism: upturned walking stick as an aid to locomotion. Arch Phys Med Rehabil 68:380, 1987
36. Bagley S, Kelly B, Tunnicliffe N, Turnbull GI, Walker JM: The effect of visual cues on the gait of independently mobile Parkinson's patients. Physiotherapy 77:415, 1991

6 | Cognitive Deficits

John D. Fisk
Susan E. Doble

The clinical diagnosis of Parkinson's disease (PD) is based on the obvious impairments of movement that are the signs of this disorder. However, James Parkinson's original observation of "the senses and intellects being uninjured"[1] has been challenged by more recent research that recognizes the existence of cognitive deficits in association with PD.[2] The majority of research concerning the cognitive deficits of PD has been limited to either describing the prevalence of generalized cognitive deficits in the PD population or describing the nature of specific deficits of cognitive ability in smaller samples of PD patients. Much remains to be learned about the cognitive deficits of PD, and continued research will be necessary for understanding the nature of these deficits and their impact on the PD patient's life. Debate continues over issues such as the prevalence of generalized or specific cognitive deficits, the influence of motor impairments on cognitive test performance, and the ability to identify a specific syndrome of deficits associated with PD. For the healthcare worker attempting to understand how cognitive impairments can interfere with the therapeutic process in PD, interpreting the varied theoretical and methodologic approaches and the inconsistencies in findings in the research literature can be extremely challenging.

This chapter will review the research into the cognitive deficits that have been described in association with PD. The first sections of the chapter will examine the issue of generalized cognitive impairment or *dementia,* its prevalence in PD, its association with disorders of mood, and its distinctiveness from other neurodegenerative processes such as Alzheimer's disease. The remaining sections will examine the evidence for specific cognitive deficits in PD. The vast majority of studies that have described the presence of specific cognitive deficits in PD have utilized clinical neuropsychologic or experimental methods that may not have obvious relevance to the healthcare worker involved in therapy with PD patients. Nevertheless, by being aware of the potential deficits that individual patients may exhibit, the healthcare worker will be in a better position to recognize those deficits when they appear in the course of therapy and to anticipate challenges to the rehabilitative process that will arise as a result of these deficits.

GENERALIZED BEHAVIORAL DEFICITS IN PARKINSON'S DISEASE

The Concept of Subcortical Dementia in Parkinson's Disease

The term most often applied to a generalized decline in cognitive ability is *dementia*. Although in recent years there has been considerable clarification of the criteria for applying this term to a patient with a suspected decline in cognitive function,[3] it is important to recognize that the term dementia should not be considered a diagnosis. Rather, it should be thought of as a term that reflects a group of symptoms of cognitive decline as well as a decline in ability that is of functional significance. It is also important to recognize that the presence of dementia is not determined on the basis of a score on a test of mental status. In a number of healthcare settings, the role of completing a mental-status questionnaire will fall to one of the healthcare professionals on the treatment team. It is important for these individuals to recognize the limitations of the information they obtain from the patient and to realize that they are unlikely to have sufficient information to "diagnose" the patient as suffering from dementia. The central feature of dementia is impairment of memory, which is rarely assessed sufficiently by mental status scales. Although impairments of other cognitive abilities are also required before the term dementia can be applied to a patient, the exact nature of these impairments may be quite variable and may be difficult to appreciate through casual observation.

The term *subcortical dementia* was originally used to describe intellectual and cognitive changes associated with progressive supranuclear palsy.[4] As with PD, progressive supranuclear palsy is a neurodegenerative process that affects subcortical structures and results in severe impairments of motor ability. Although PD and progressive supranuclear palsy share many symptoms, progressive supranuclear palsy does not respond to dopamine replacement therapy, and has additional oculamotor symptoms.[5] Followong the initial description of subcortical dementia, a similar syndrome of cognitive decline was described in association with PD.[6,7] Subsequently, the term subcortical dementia has been applied to a number of other disorders, such as Huntington's disease,[2] that are characterized by pathology of subcortical structures and that have associated cognitive impairments. Widespread use of the term subcortical dementia has not been without controversy, however. To date, there is by no means a consensus in the scientific and medical literature regarding its use.

Despite controversy over the appropriateness and use of the term subcortical dementia, there does appear to be some general understanding of what this term implies. To some extent, this agreement is based on the clinical features

Table 6-1. Clinical Features of Cortical and Subcortical Dementia

	Cortical	Subcortical
Memory impairment	+	+
Aphasia	+	−
Apraxia	+	−
Agnosia	+	−
Slowed information processing	?	+
Mood disturbance/Personality Change	?	+

that distinguish "subcortical dementia" from "cortical dementia," a term that is usually taken to mean the cognitive deficits associated with Alzheimer's disease (Table 6-1). Memory disturbances are a required feature of both cortical and subcortical dementia. The features that are typically considered to reflect subcortical dementia include the absence of aphasia, apraxia, and agnosia and the prominence of slowed information processing and mood or personality disturbances. It is very important to recognize, however, that these proposed differentiating features have almost never had clear operational definitions, and that there has been a notable lack of good comparative studies of various diagnostic groups.[8] Nevertheless, despite the questionable validity of the term subcortical dementia, it has made its way into the clinical terminology of PD. Although many would argue about the appropriateness of describing the cognitive deficits associated with PD as a subcortical dementia, most would agree that any healthcare worker who sees a reasonable number of patients with PD will almost certainly be faced with patients who meet the recognized diagnostic criteria for dementia.[3]

The Prevalence of Dementia in Parkinson's Disease

Most clinicians and researchers who have experience with PD will agree that dementia is an important clinical issue even though estimates of its prevalence can vary considerably. This variation reflects a number of factors, including the criteria used for the presence of dementia, the age of the population with which one is in contact, and the clinical practice in which one is engaged. Generalization of the data from any one study is impossible, and it can be difficult to interpret data from early studies, many of which were conducted before 1980, because of inconsistencies in patient diagnoses and in the criteria for the presence of dementia. This has resulted in reported prevalence rates that have varied from 20 percent of PD patients with dementia of sufficient severity to require assistance for activities of daily living to 93 percent of PD patients with evidence of some degree of cognitive impairment.[6] Although a precise estimate of the prevalence of dementia in PD remains elusive, dementia is more prevalent in patients with PD than in appropriately matched controls from the general medical population.[9]

In a comparative study of patients with PD, Alzheimer's disease, and Huntington's disease, Mayeaux and colleagues[10] reported a prevalence of

38.6 percent for dementia in their PD sample (22 of 57 patients), while 60 percent of their patients with Huntington's disease (12 of 20) and 100 percent of those with Alzheimer's disease (46 of 46) were considered to be demented. Although their diagnostic criteria for dementia were consistent with currently accepted criteria, actual testing of cognitive functioning was limited to a modified version of a simple mental-status test. They divided their group of PD subjects into three levels of functional impairment, based largely on ratings of activities of daily living, and found that the more functionally impaired subjects were older, had a longer duration of symptoms, and had lower scores on the test of mental status. Thus, even though the mean age of the PD subjects in this study was only 64.4 years, the findings suggested that dementia may be a more significant issue with elderly and more functionally impaired PD patients.

An even lower prevalence of dementia in PD patients was found in a later study in which Mayeaux and colleagues[11] reviewed the medical records of a consecutive series of 339 patients with PD over an 18-month interval. Of this sample, only 10.9 percent were judged to meet their criteria for dementia. Unfortunately, although mental-status testing was reportedly completed for all patients, neuropsychologic assessments were available for an unspecified and presumably small number. Once again, dementia was associated with increased age and increased severity of symptoms. In addition, the prevalence odds ratio for dementia was found to be 3.75 times greater for patients with onset of PD after age 70.

A longitudinal study by Ebmeier et al.[12] of a more elderly sample of PD patients (median age = 75.3 years) also suggested that the presence of dementia in PD is related to age and symptom severity. Follow-up of a cohort of 127 patients with PD for a 3 1/2-year period revealed that 23.6 percent of the patients met the criteria for dementia at follow-up. As did Mayeaux et al.,[11] Ebmeier et al.[12] reported that demented patients had more severe symptoms, were older, and had a later age of onset of symptoms. Logistic regression analyses demonstrated the value of age and symptom severity in predicting the presence of dementia at follow-up; unfortunately, age of symptom onset was not included as an independent variable in the analyses they reported. Other studies have also noted a higher prevalence of dementia in PD patients with onset of symptoms in their later years.[13] Despite the consistency of these findings, dementia is not limited to PD patients with a late onset of symptoms. Regardless of the age of onset of symptoms, the reported prevalence rates for dementia in PD patients exceed the estimates of the prevalence of dementia in community-based epidemiologic studies.[14] Thus, from the standpoint of therapeutic intervention, one cannot assume the presence or absence of dementia for an individual patient, regardless of the patient's age or level of disease severity.

Despite the variation in the reported prevalence rates for dementia in PD, continued efforts to define precisely its prevalence appear to be unnecessary at present. It is already clear that a decline in cognitive abilities is an important issue for a significant proportion of PD patients even though this proportion of the population may be smaller than that with other neurodegenerative disorders, such as Alzheimer's disease. While some PD patients may exhibit a number of specific cognitive deficits, they may not meet the criteria for a variety of reasons. First, the term dementia implies the presence of cognitive deficits that pose clear functional limitations. In a PD patient who already exhibits neurologic motor signs that pose obvious and severe functional limitations, the functional impact of some cognitive deficits may be very difficult to estimate. This clinical presentation of the PD patient is in stark contrast to the presentation of patients with Alzheimer's disease who, by definition, have dementia and only minimal neurologic signs. Second, memory impairment, the essential feature of dementia, reflects impairment of a complex process. Although some memory impairments will be apparent on casual observation, more subtle deficits may be evident only with thorough, quantitative testing that is often impractical for population-based studies. Third, one must necessarily expect that the prevalence of dementia will be reduced in PD relative to conditions such as Alzheimer's disease, since the criteria for dementia include features that are considered to reflect cortical dysfunction (e.g., aphasia, apraxia, agnosia) and are not typically associated with the cognitive deficits found in PD.

Restricting the scope of future investigations of cognitive functioning in PD to the global concept of dementia may be of limited scientific and clinical value because of the variety of specific cognitive deficits that PD patients may exhibit. Even though the prevalence of dementia may not be exceedingly high in PD, the prevalence of specific cognitive deficits may be much higher.[15] Because specific deficits of cognitive functioning may be quite variable in their nature and severity, however, the question that must be asked is whether they are likely to have significant impact on those functional abilities that are the target of the rehabilitative process. Rather than attempting to identify the prevalence of dementia in PD, it seems more appropriate to examine the cognitive deficits that characterize PD, the prevalence of these deficits, the relationship of these deficits to other clinical factors, and the impact of these deficits on the lives of patients with PD.

Mood Disorders in Parkinson's Disease

A complicating feature of the questions surrounding the cognitive changes associated with PD is the issue of depression. Depression has been reported to be common in PD patients,[16] and it is recognized that cognitive changes associated with depression can result in a presentation similar to that of dementia, particularly in elderly patients.[17] The term *pseudodementia* has occasionally been used to describe the cognitive changes associated with depression, and Caine[17] pointed out the similarities between the cognitive deficits associated with the concepts of pseudodementia and subcortical dementia. Some of these similarities include slowed performance of motor tasks as well as slowness of thought. This latter problem is analogous to the slowed processing of information or *bradyphrenia* that has been considered to be associated with PD (see the section on Speed of Information Processing).

Two major questions have been asked about depression in PD. First, does a consistent relationship exist between depression and cognitive deficits in PD?

The answer to this question continues to remain unclear. A second, related question is whether depression is endogenous and therefore reflects the underlying neuropathologic process in PD, or whether it represents a reaction to the physical, cognitive, and social disabilities imposed by PD. The answer to this second question appears to be that both of these possibilities exist.[18] In a retrospective chart review of 339 cases of PD, Sano and colleagues[19] reported a 51 percent prevalence for depression, a 10.9 percent prevalence for dementia, and a 5.4 percent prevalence for the coexistence of depression and dementia. Although these figures suggest relative independence of these behavioral disorders, a prospective study of 115 patients revealed evidence of a specific neurotransmitter abnormality (decreased serotonin metabolite levels in the cerebrospinal fluid) only in those patients with coexisting depression and dementia. Based on this finding, Sano et al. suggested that the coexistence of depression and dementia in PD represent a distinct syndrome in which a common biochemical deficit underlies both behavioral disorders. It must be remembered, however, that this appeared to be the case for only a very small proportion of their PD sample.

Other studies have failed to find a relationship between depression and specific cognitive impairments in PD,[20] and have not supported the concept of a common underlying cause for depression and cognitive deficits in the disease. Starkenstein and colleagues[21] found an inverse relationship between the age of symptom onset and the prevalence of depression, which is in direct contrast to the positive relationship between age of symptom onset and prevalence of dementia that others have found. Even when matched for the duration of disease, PD patients with onset of symptoms before age 55 were more likely to meet diagnostic criteria for depression[3] than those with symptom onset after age 55. Although this finding might lead one to conclude that depression in PD must represent a reaction to the disability imposed by the disease, Starkenstein and colleagues[22] also provided evidence for specific neural dysfunction in association with depression in PD. Using positron emission tomography (PET), they found that reduced metabolic activity in the inferior and orbital frontal regions of the cortex was associated with the presence and severity of depressive symptoms. Although these authors suggested that this pattern of metabolic abnormality is distinct from that seen in association with dementia in PD, they did not present data supporting this suggestion. Although the findings of Starkenstein et al.[21,22] suggest a dissociation between depression and dementia in PD, they imply that the neural dysfunction is the underlying cause of depression in PD.

Findings in keeping with the possibility that depression in PD arises as a reaction to a chronic, disabling illness have also been presented, however. Brown et al.[23] performed a prospective study of 132 PD patients that employed self-report measures of mood. Although the same proportion of the sample (36/132) met the criteria for depression on initial testing and follow-up, only 21 patients met the criteria for depression on both occasions. Self-reported depression correlated only modestly with disability in activities of daily living ($r = .45$, .41) on both occasions. Furthermore, changes in the ratings of depression and disability showed even less of a relationship to each other ($r = .16$). Thus, the relationship between disability and depression in PD is by no means simple. For some PD patients, depression may be a constant and stable feature of their symptoms. Perhaps in these patients, depressive symptoms arise as a direct result of the neuropathologic process of PD. For other patients, depressive symptoms appear to be related to a number of factors, which may include the patient's age, absolute level of physical disability, and rate of progression of disability. Perhaps a more important issue than the absolute level of disability or rate of change of disability, however, is the patient's perception of the importance or significance of a change in functional ability for the patient's own life. As with all chronic, disabling diseases, the impact of PD on the patient's mood must be considered on an individual basis, since the significance of physical disabilities and a change in functional limitations will depend on a number of factors that may be unique to the individual patient. It is quite possible for a patient who remains functional to be more depressed than a more disabled patient. The healthcare worker must consider what the disease means to each patient in terms of lifestyle, future goals, and the patient's self-perception as a competent and worthy individual. Therapeutic goals must also take into account these factors to ensure that the goals are meaningful to the patient.

Research to date indicates that depression is an important issue in the healthcare of PD patients. As with the issue of dementia, each patient must be considered to be an individual. The meaning or significance of PD will be different for each patient, and the healthcare worker should not assume that the patient either will or will not experience symptoms of depression. Because of the potential impact of depression on attempts at therapeutic intervention, it is important that healthcare workers recognize the existence of depression in their patients when it occurs. This can be difficult, since many of the symptoms of PD mimic those of depression. These symptoms include the lack of variation in facial expression, the slowness of movement, and the apparent slowness of thought. The inability of PD patients to vary the pitch and loudness of their speech production and their lack of facial expression limit the range of affect that they can display. This in turn makes it difficult for the healthcare worker to interpret a patient's mood. For some patients, depression does appear to reflect the underlying neuropathologic process of PD, and they may therefore not respond to behavioral interventions aimed at improving mood. In such instances, healthcare workers may find that improvements in functional status have no effect on the mood of the patient.

Significant gaps between functional ability and performance, and a failure to respond to therapy, can reflect either cognitive deficits or depression, making differentiation of these possibilities difficult. Although it may be much easier to assume that treatment failures reflect the presence of dementia, it is always better to assume that they reflect depression, until proven otherwise by the patient. Depression is amenable to either pharmacologic or psychotherapeutic intervention, whereas there is no treatment for the cognitive deficits of PD. Although depression and dementia both have an increased prevalence in PD, it is important to recognize that they appear to coexist in a small proportion of the PD population. When patients with presumed depression fail to respond to treatment, further assessment is required to differentiate between depression and dementia. As with the assessment of dementia, depression cannot be diagnosed on the basis of any one simple measure, such as a self-report mood inventory, and a referral to another healthcare professional should be considered whenever this issue arises.

SPECIFIC COGNITIVE DEFICITS IN PARKINSON'S DISEASE

The studies described above have examined the cognitive deficits associated with PD in the context of the generalized decline in ability associated with dementia only. The following sections describe research that has focused on specific cognitive abilities in PD. The organization of the discussion partly reflects the typical manner in which neuropsychologists group cognitive abilities in accordance with their functional significance and neuroanatomic correlates.

Memory Impairments in Parkinson's Disease

Findings of memory impairment associated with PD are implied in all of the studies that have examined dementia in PD, since memory impairment of functional significance is a requirement of the accepted diagnostic criteria for dementia.[3] Memory is by no means a simple construct, however, and a tremendous body of literature has been devoted to the study of memory in psychology. Therefore, it is important to consider whether there is a pattern of memory impairment in PD that is distinct from that in other neurologic conditions, and whether this pattern has neuroanatomic, biochemical, and functional significance.

One of the most challenging aspects of the psychological assessment of memory is the quantitative assessment of remote memory. Since remote memory represents information that has been acquired over one's lifetime, individual variation in personal experience has posed significant problems for the construction of standardized instruments for assessing it. The most thorough attempt to assess remote memory in PD has been reported by Sagar and colleagues,[24] who conducted a comparative study of patients with PD, Alzheimer's disease, and normal controls. Remote memory for both public and personal events was examined with a variety of procedures, but of particular importance was that the content of memory and the dating of past events were examined separately. Although the patients with Alzheimer's disease were by far the most severely impaired on all tests of memory, the pattern that emerged for the PD patients was one of adequate memory of the content of remote events but a relative deficiency in dating these events. Even when recalling personal events, the PD patients demonstrated an impaired ability to recall "time-specific" events. This specific impairment of temporal dating of past events by the PD subjects was in contrast to the more severe and global impairments of memory for both content and date by the Alzheimer's disease patients. Although the memory impairment of the Alzheimer's disease patients was clearly related to their degree of dementia as measured by a mental-status scale, a relatively selective impairment of dating capacity was apparent in PD patients both with and without evidence of cognitive decline on this simple screening measure.

In contrast to the limited number of assessment instruments for remote memory that have been developed by psychologists, they have been quite prolific in generating instruments for assessing the ability to learn new information. A study by El-Awar and colleagues[25] is representative of the findings that have typically been reported for PD patients on such tests. As in the study of Sagar et al.,[24] El-Awar et al. used a comparative approach to examine 12 individuals with PD, 10 with Alzheimer's disease, and 12 normal controls. Their task was a paired-associates learning test in which the subjects were required to learn 10 pairs of randomly paired words over 10 learning trials. Although they separated the PD subjects into two subgroups without statistical justification, their general comparisons of the PD and control subjects are typical of the memory-test performance of PD patients. As a group, PD patients were less able than controls to learn the word pairings. Some PD patients appeared to differ little from controls in this capacity, whereas others more closely approximated the almost total failure of learning that the patients with Alzheimer's disease demonstrated. Despite this general difficulty in initial learning, however, the PD group did not differ from the control group in their ability to retain whatever information they had learned after a delay interval of 1 hour. Furthermore, after 1 hour, their ability to recognize the word association in a forced-choice situation did not differ from that of the controls.

Recognition of the memory impairments that may be associated with PD is of considerable importance for the healthcare worker. Perhaps the most damaging assumption that can be made is that the patient is not trying to learn a new task or skill. Studies of new learning by PD patients have usually revealed a decreased capacity or slowed rate of initial learning of new information. Thus, increased time and effort may be required of the patient, particularly for tasks that involve the recall of verbal instructions. However, PD patients do not appear to suffer from an excessive rate of forgetting whatever information has been learned. Although a deficient ability to retrieve information from memory is usually evident when PD patients are asked to recall previously presented material, they are able to benefit from cues to aid their memory retrieval. Thus, the use of simple memory aids such as calendars and appointment books may prove useful to some PD patients. The increased use of contextual cues, such as learning to perform a task in the environment in which it will typically be performed, may also facilitate new learning. For most PD patients, the possibility for continued adaptation to new challenges should exist, although this possibility is greatly limited for some patients.

Conceptual Ability (Frontal Lobe Functioning)

Despite the lack of significant pathologic changes in the cerebral cortex of PD patients, disturbances in cortical functioning have been implied from a number of neuropsychologic findings. In particular, the loss of ascending dopaminergic input to the cortex has been implicated in a number of cognitive deficits that typify frontal-lope dysfunction. One of the best known examples of this was reported by Lees and Smith,[26] who examined a group of 30 relatively young PD patients (less than 65 years of age) with a recent onset of symptoms (less than 5 years) and only mild disability. Their sample of PD patients did not differ from age-matched control subjects on tests of general intellectual ability or on forced-choice recognition memory tests. Significant differences were evident, however, on a test of deductive reasoning ability that requires the subject to use feedback provided by the examiner to identify and alternate between response strategies for sorting cards into categories. The PD subjects demonstrated an inability to change their manner of categorization despite repeated feedback from the examiner that their responses were incorrect. This resulted in a high proportion of the type of errors that are referred to as *perseverative* in the neuropsychologic literature. Such inflexibility or "stickiness" in thinking is considered typical of patients with frontal-lobe dysfunction, on the basis of studies of patients with localized cortical excisions for the treatment of intractable epilepsy.[27] However, the presence of this type of cognitive deficit in PD patients without cortical pathologic changes has been implied by studies of PD patients in the early stages of the disease[28] and has been confirmed by autopsy findings in selected PD patients.[29]

The types of cognitive deficits that are typically associated with frontal-lobe dysfunction have been difficult for neuropsychologists to operationalize. Similarly, the implications of these types of deficits for everyday activities can be very difficult to estimate. Specialized neuropsychologic tests can make it possible to identify and quantify such cognitive deficits, but their effects on the performance of everyday activities can be more subtle. For example, PD patients may experience difficulties in using assistive devices to perform routine activities and may have difficulty in adapting to modifications in the environment that have been designed to improve mobility. They may also demonstrate impaired social judgement and reasoning in the form of an inability to appreciate alternative solutions to problems. Such patients may be unable to appreciate the subtle social cues that form the basis for normal interaction. Consequently, they may require more explicit and overt guidance, particularly when attempting to develop new behaviors. Unfortunately, such difficulties in cognitive functioning are often viewed as either stubbornness or uncooperative behavior on the part of the patient, or as inflexibility due to aging in more elderly patients. These viewpoints will jeopardize the patient's therapeutic relationship with healthcare workers, as well as the relationship with family and other care providers. It is critical for healthcare workers, family members and other caregivers to recognize and appreciate these behavioral changes as a feature of the disease process. Since treatment is unlikely to have an effect on these behaviors, the healthcare worker must consider their potential impact when setting therapeutic goals. Rather than attempting to teach the patient new skills, the practice of building on established patterns of behavior may enable the patient to maintain a greater level of independence. While assistive devices may make some behaviors easier to perform, the healthcare worker must consider whether the process of adapting to such devices will be more frustrating and stressful than helpful.

Spatial Abilities

Impaired performance of tasks that require spatial abilities has commonly been reported in neuropsychologic studies of PD, and a very high prevalence of impaired spatial ability has been reported for PD patients.[30] The existence of spatial impairments in PD has not been without controversy, however,[30,31] and a failure to find significant spatial impairments in selected tasks performed by PD patients has also been reported.[33,34] The concept of spatial abilities is quite broad, and a wide variety of tasks have been employed to examine this general class of abilities. Impairment of spatial ability is usually considered to represent "difficulty in appreciating the relative position of stimulus-objects in space, difficulty in integrating those objects into a coherent framework, and difficulty in performing mental operations involving spatial concepts."[36] As with most of the neuropsychologic literature on PD, comparisons between studies on spatial abilities is often difficult. For the most part, however, the discrepant findings that have been reported can often be explained by differences in the operational definition of spatial behaviors, differences in the choice of experimental tasks, and differences in the patient population or selection criteria.

One difficulty in interpreting the literature on spatial impairments in PD arises because the tasks used to examine these abilities are often time-limited and may place considerable demands on efficient ocular motor scanning ability or may require complex motor responses. This raises serious questions about the extent to which impaired performance on these tasks is related to a specific impairment of spatial abilities. Impaired performance by PD patients has been noted on relatively simple spatial tasks, such as setting the angle of a moveable rod to match a model under either visual or tactile guidance.[36,37] However, even such simple tasks are not free from the potential influence of impaired motor abilities. Furthermore, scores on such tests often fail to correlate with clinical measures of visual perceptual discrimination that do not require accurate motor responses. As a result, impairments of spatial abilities and impairments of motor abilities can be difficult to distinguish in the neuropsychologic test performance of PD patients.

As with all tests of cognitive abilities for PD patients, considerable variability exists between individual patients in spatial task performance, and overly broad generalizations have little scientific or clinical utility. Figure 6-1 illustrates the variability of the performance of two patients with PD who were asked to copy a complex geometric drawing, a typical neuropsychologic test of constructional ability. Although the effects of tremor are obvious in the drawing on the

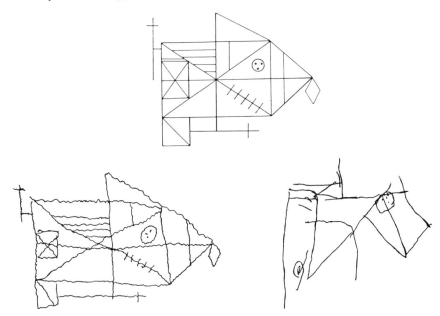

Fig. 6-1. Examples of attempts to copy a complex geometric figure by two patients with PD. The drawing on the left illustrates the effects of the subject's tremor. The drawing on the right demonstrates the spatial disorganization that characterizes constructional apraxia.

left of the figure, it is equally obvious that this patient was able to reproduce correctly the spatial organization of the figure. In contrast, the other patient, who demonstrated less evidence of tremor and bradykinesia, demonstrated considerable difficulty in reproducing the spatial relationships of the component items and produced a figure that typifies a constructional apraxia.

Despite the possible contribution of motor impairments to impaired spatial test performance, deficient performance on spatial reasoning tasks that have minimal motor requirements has been demonstrated in PD. In a comparative study, Huber, Shuttleworth and Fredenberg[38] found that groups of PD patients and Alzheimer's disease patients who were matched on the basis of mental-status scale scores were both impaired on spatial tasks relative to control subjects. Surprisingly, however, when the PD and Alzheimer's disease groups were compared, the PD group performed less well on a task of spatial reasoning and better on a constructional task with high motor demands. Although generalization from this study is difficult because the PD sample was selected on the basis of the presence of dementia, the findings nevertheless suggest that there is some basis for considering that a specific impairment of spatial ability accompanies PD.

Perhaps the most thorough investigation of the spatial impairments of a more representative sample of PD patients was done by Boller et al.[35] They employed tasks characterized by either minimal motor demands (visual spatial) or significant motor demands (visual motor) to examine the performance of PD patients and control subjects. Factor analysis of the subjects' test scores generally supported their a priori classification of these tests. However, even though Boller and colleagues were able to demonstrate that PD patients with relatively mild signs of motor dysfunction were impaired relative to normal controls on spatial tests with minimal motor requirements, they were unable to demonstrate a specific impairment of visual-spatial or visual-motor ability for their PD patients. They suggested that PD patients with more advanced disease were more impaired on both visual-spatial and visual-motor tests, although this suggestion was not supported by statistically significant group differences. They also pointed out that correlational analyses failed to reveal any relationship between their estimates of IQ or depressed mood and either visual-spatial or visual-motor ability. However, data in support of this claim was not presented.

Despite the inconsistencies in the existing literature on the spatial abilities of PD patients, there does exist a body of evidence that PD patients are impaired in the performance of spatial tasks. Impairments of visual-spatial abilities appear to be somewhat independent from the more global concept of dementia, since impaired spatial task performance has been demonstrated in PD patients who are only mildly affected. However, the specific nature of visual-spatial deficits in PD and their implications for daily activities has yet to be fully described. In part, the visual-spatial and visual-motor deficits that are revealed by neuropsychologic tests probably reflect a more generalized deficiency in the ability of PD patients to integrate perception and motor behavior. No typical human activity can be considered either purely perceptual or purely motor, and it is not surprising that the behavioral impairments of PD reflect both perceptual and motor deficits. It has also been recognized for some time that additional sensory cues, such as a visual grid on the floor, can facilitate effective motor behavior by PD patients. The spatial impairments of PD patients that are revealed through neuropsychologic testing may reflect only one component of a generalized deficit in the ability to integrate visual-perceptual information with the planning and execution of a motor act. Thus, when attempting to improve the motor functioning of the PD patient, the healthcare worker must also consider the visual-spatial requirements of the relevant behaviors. Performing self-care and instrumental activities of daily living, particularly when using a cane or walker, involves considerable spatial skill in estimating the sizes and angles of objects and spaces in the environment. Therapy that focuses only on developing skill capacities, such as strength and range of motion, will be of limited value. The ability to function within a normal environment requires reaching, turning, positioning, and navigating one's body in relation to furnishings, objects and other individuals, all of which require spatial abilities.

Language

Language has often been considered the exclusive domain of cortical brain function. In part, this may reflect the bias of considering language as a class of behavior unique to humans, coupled with the opinion that subcortical brain structures represent a lower order of evolutionary development. However, studies of patients with focal lesions of vascular origin have demonstrated that basal ganglionic structures are intimately involved in language.[39] Despite this, the aphasic syndromes resulting from focal lesions of the basal ganglia are not a feure of PD, and the impact of PD on language functioning remains less clear. Although aphasia is not evident, dysarthria and dysphonia are very prevalent and are often early manifestions of PD. Their presence has typically been attributed to the characteristic motor deficits of PD rather than to any deficit of cognition.[40]

Darkins et al.[41] have supported the argument for a speech-production deficit in PD in their study of the comprehension and expression of the linguistic and affective information conveyed by changes in the pitch, loudness, and duration of speech sounds (prosody). On the basis of intact performance by PD patients on routine tests for aphasia and on a test of prosodic comprehension, Darkins and colleagues argued that the linguistic system remains intact in PD. Since none of their subjects fell below the suggested cutoff score for dementia on a test of mental status, they also argued against any association between prosodic output deficits and dementia. Correlational analysis failed to reveal any significant relationship between ratings of depression and measures of prosodic production, and suggested that a disorder of mood could not account for the lack of prosodic output in the speech of PD patients. As noted in the previous section on mood disorders, the lack of prosody in the PD patient's speech makes it difficult to interpret the patient's mood. At times, this lack of expression can make it difficult to tell whether a patient has made a joke or an inappropriate comment. Although increased experience with the patient will typically reveal individual cues that can assist in interpreting the patient's mood, corroborative information about the patient's personality, from reliable sources, can also be informative.

Although deficient prosodic output is a clear feature of PD, the presence of other deficiencies of language ability has been suggested for at least some portion of the population of PD patients. Matison et al.[42] noted that a number of their PD patients had difficulty with a test that requires the naming of a standard set of line drawings.[43] This word-finding difficulty was found to be related to disease severity in their PD patients. Word-finding difficulties have since been noted by others as well. Matison et al. suggested that such difficulties represent a deficiency of "semantic retrieval" that reflects an impairment in planning or shifting cognitive set, similar to the impairments resulting from frontal-lobe dysfunction. Beatty and Monson[44] conducted a more extensive examination of language abilities in situations that required word production for semantic, visual, or rhyming cues. They found that PD patients who had impaired naming for standard drawings also had impaired word-finding under all other conditions, indicating that this problem reflects a generalized disorder of language that cannot be explained by visual-perceptual difficulties or by a generalized slowing of response. Although only one of the eight patients included in their "impaired naming" group scored below the typical cutoff score for dementia on a test of mental status, it is not clear that the language disturbances in PD can generally be distinguished from the concept of dementia.

When Matison et al. employed an operational definition of dementia that was based on neuropsychologic test performance rather than a mental status test, 7 of the 8 PD patients with impaired naming and 5 of the 17 PD patients with intact naming met criteria for dementia. Thus, while the language output deficits of PD appear to be early features of PD that are related to the other characteristic motor signs of this disorder, impaired access and retrieval of linguistic information appears to be a later manifestation of more generalized cognitive decline in PD.

Speed of Information Processing

While slowing of motor behavior is one of the hallmark symptoms of PD, the issue of whether an analogous slowing of the mental processing of information also occurs in PD remains controversial. As noted earlier, some have used the term bradyphrenia to emphasize the perceived similarities between performance on tests of cognitive processing and the slowed motor abilities (bradykinesia) of PD patients. However, the operational definition of this term has been quite vague, and the neuropsychologic tests that have been employed to examine this issue have varied from tests of vigilance and sustained attention[45] to tests such as the expedited naming of objects in an embedded figures test.[46] No simple relationship has been demonstrated between bradykinesia and bradyphrenia. Some have suggested that slowed cognitive processing in PD is related to altered norepinephrine metabolism rather than dopaminergic dysfunction.[45] Others, however, who have argued for dysfunction of nondopaminergic systems, acknowledge that "it may be naive to attribute such a subtle and complex symptom as cognitive slowing to the dysfunction of a single type of neurotransmitter."[46]

The concept of cognitive slowing in PD is compelling because of the qualitative features of the way in which PD patients perform many tests of cognitive ability. Indeed, one is quite often left with the impression that this slowing of performance cannot be solely explained by the slowing of motor responses. However, clear evidence for slowed cognitive processing remains elusive. To evaluate the time required for "central" processing of information, as opposed to the time required to execute a motor act, it is essential that all motor aspects of a task be controlled. Thus, the best means of examining the speed of cognitive processing is to compare the performance of an individual subject on tests that require the analysis of differing amounts of information but involve the same behavioral response. Typically, comparisons of subjects' performances of simple and complex reaction-time (RT) tasks have been used for this purpose. However, such paradigms, have generally failed to reveal an increased difference between PD and control subjects on complex RT tasks that have increased information processing demands.[33,47,48] Thus, although PD patients are slower to respond to the onset of a stimulus, they have not been shown to have a disproportionate increase in RT if asked to respond only when certain types of stimuli are presented. It has been argued that RT studies have failed to support the construct of bradyphrenia because the relatively simple nature of these tasks does not require the same degree of information processing required in the neuropsychologic measures on which bradyphrenia is evident.[48] However, it must be acknowledged that the most adequately controlled studies have failed to support the construct of bradyphrenia. The resistance of some to abandon the concept of bradyphrenia in PD may in part arise from the viewpoint that slowing of information processing is a feature of subcortical dementia, and that subcortical dementia is a valid way of conceptualizing the cognitive deficits associated with PD. However, the best available evidence suggests that slowed cognitive processing of information, independent of the programming and execution of motor behavior, is not characteristic of, or at least not specific to, PD.

Attention

Although *attention* is a common lay term, the concept of attention in psychological research has been difficult to define and operationalize. As with the concept of spatial abilities discussed earlier, many varied tasks have been employed in the study of attention in PD, and diverse findings have been reported. While some have hypothesized that impaired attention is a central feature of the cognitive deficits in PD, others have reported a failure to find evidence of impaired attention. To some extent, these discrepancies in the literature appear to reflect variations in the level of difficulty or complexity of the tasks that have been studied. Despite these discrepancies, this approach, which employs a methodology based on models of information processing from cognitive psychological research, seems to hold the most promise for the development of an understanding of the effects of PD on cognitive processes.

One of the most influential approaches to the study of attention was developed by Posner.[49] The paradigm that he developed involved an RT procedure in which a cue for the probable location of a target in the peripheral visual field (left versus right) was indicated before its appearance by a cue (arrow) presented in the central visual field. By comparing the subjects' RTs under conditions in which the central cue correctly predicted the probable location of the target (valid cue) with their reaction times under conditions in which the central cue provided no information (neutral cue) or in which the cue provided an incorrect indication of the target location (invalid cue), Posner was able to operationalize and quantify the process of attention-shifting to different portions of the visual field. To ensure that this shift in attention was independent of the process of moving the eyes, the subjects were required to maintain their gaze on the central position even after the cue had been provided. Posner and co-workers[50] then applied this same technique to the study of PD patients before and after pharmacologic treatment. Although they found improvements in overall RT following pharmacologic treatment, no changes were noted in the measures of attention shifting. Since no control group was included in this study, however, it could not be determined whether the PD patients suffered from any impairment of attention. A comparative study of PD patients and matched elderly control subjects was done by Wright et al.[51] using the same paradigm. Although the PD patients demonstrated the expected slowness in their overall RTs, they were as capable as the control subjects of improving their performance when provided with valid central cues. Surprisingly, Wright et al. found that PD patients demonstrated less of an adverse effect on the speed of attention-shifting when provided with an invalid cue. Thus, studies using Posner's paradigm raise questions about whether any deficit in attention is associated with PD, although the generalization of these results to other paradigms must be examined.

Goodrich and colleagues[52] reported findings somewhat similar to those of Wright et al.[51] in a comparative study of simple and complex RTs for PD and control subjects. Their study differed from the other studies in that their paradigm required responses to a tactile stimulus rather than a visual target. Once again, overall RTs were much lower for the PD patients under all conditions, although Goodrich et al. found that the normal increase in RT when a complex rather than a simple response was required was not as marked for the PD group. They acknowledged others had previously made this finding, but they were also able to demonstrate that the introduction of a distractor task (oral reading) had minimal effects on the RTs of the PD patients despite producing a significant increase in the RTs of the control subjects. In many ways, this finding appears analogous to the reduced adverse effect of invalid cuing in Posner's paradigm as demonstrated by Wright et al.[51] The relative improvement of PD patients' RT performance under conditions of slightly increased task complexity suggests that either PD facilitates cognitive processing or that it confers a specific disadvantage under simple task conditions. Clearly, it is the latter interpretation that is more likely. Goodrich et al.[52] interpreted this selective impairment of simple RT performance by PD patients as evidence of an inability to recruit the attention-enhancing resources that are normally available in situations requiring simple responses to expected stimuli.

A deficiency in the ability to recruit attentional resources for the performance of simple tasks seems to be a plausible feature of PD. However, studies that have used much more complex tasks have suggested a very different pattern of impairment for PD patients. Brown and Marsden[53] hypothesized that PD patients demonstrate a deficient ability to use "internal attentional control" to direct their behavior, despite having an intact ability to utilize external cues for guidance. To explore this hypothesis they utilized a modified version of the Stroop task, in which the subject is required to respond to the relevant attribute of a word written in colored ink (e.g., the word "red" written in green ink). Subjects are asked to either read the word or identify the color of the ink, based on a cue provided by the experimenter. In their version of this task, Brown and Marsden provided cues either before each stimulus (external cue) or before blocks of trials. In this latter condition the subjects were required to rely on their memory for the appropriate attribute (internal cue). Although the presence or absence of explicit cues before each trial had no effect on the control subjects' performance, the PD patients were significantly slower for the internal cue condition. Using the model of attention proposed by Norman and Shallice[54] and modified by Baddely,[55] Brown and Marsden[53] suggested that the PD patients' impaired performance reflects the overloading of a limited-capacity "supervisory attentional system" that comes into play in situations that involve planning or decision making, performing novel or poorly learned tasks, or overcoming habitual responses. According to their hypothesis, the lack of explicit external cues for the Stroop task resulted in overloading of this "supervisory attentional system" in the PD patients. The same argument could also be applied to the types of cognitive deficits that were described in the previous section on conceptual ability and frontal-lobe functioning. The only difference between the study of Brown and Marsden[53] and those described previously may be that while they took an approach based on cognitive psychological theory, others took a clinical neuropsychologic approach based on theories of localization of brain function.

Although considerable work remains in this field of research, the cognitive neuropsychologic approach that has been used in studying the attentional process in PD appears to hold promise in providing a theoretical framework in which the varied deficits of PD patients can be understood and their discrepant performance on tasks that are presumed to examine the same cognitive ability can be interpreted. The research so far done on attentional processes fails to suggest any simple model of impairment in PD, but does provide a strong argument against the rather simple-minded notion of "bradyphrenia" or slowing of information processing. Rather, it appears that attentional deficits in PD may work at two levels. For tasks in which a simple motor reponse to an expected stimulus is required, PD patients appear to have difficulty in recruiting the additional attentional resources that are normally available to facilitate responses. In slightly more complex tasks, when such additional resources are not routinely available, the slowed responses of the PD patient may reflect only a slowing of motor responses rather than any slowing of information processing. However, under yet more complex circumstances, where responses are less obviously constrained by the physical attributes of the stimuli, the attentional capacity of the PD subject may be exceeded. Thus, the situations that will cause particular difficulty for the PD patient are those that require planning and decision making, that involve novel or poorly learned tasks, or that require the overcoming of habitual responses. In contrast, structuring and simplifying the environment in a manner that provides increased guidance about the appropriate behavior will assist in focusing the PD patient's attentional system and improve the patient's functional performance.

SUMMARY

Persons with PD are quite likely to have a reasonable understanding of the types of motor deficits they can expect with the passage of time. However, many will be quite unaware of the cognitive deficits that may accompany the disease. For some patients, it may be the cognitive deficits, rather than physical disabilities, that are the most significant limiting factor for functional activities such as driving an automobile.[56] Unless persons with PD understand that cognitive deficits may accompany the motor deficits of the disease, their inability to understand and explain what is happening to them can be extremely frightening. By explaining that these deficits are a part of the disease process, healthcare workers who are knowledgeable about the possible cognitive deficits and mood disturbances of PD will be better equipped to help the PD patient. This knowledge can, for many patients and their families, greatly facilitate their ability to adapt to the changes brought about by PD. Additionally, healthcare workers can use current knowledge of the cognitive deficits of PD to improve their manner of interacting with PD patients. One of the most important concepts in understanding the nature of cognitive deficits in PD and their impact on PD patients' lives is that each patient is a unique individual who has a personal interpretation of what PD means and how it will affect his or her lifestyle. The presence and pattern of cognitive deficits and mood disturbances will vary from one patient to another, and some patients will not experience deficits that interfere with their functional abilities.

While it is challenging for healthcare workers to interact and work with individuals who have cognitive deficits and mood disorders, it is even more challenging for the PD patient to live with these problems. To work effectively in a therapeutic role with the cognitively impaired patient, modifications in the pattern and style of interaction may be necessary. The healthcare worker may be required to slow the pace of communication so as not to overwhelm the patient. In doing so, however, it is equally important not to communicate as if the patient were a child. Even patients who meet diagnostic criteria for dementia remain individuals who are capable of thinking and feeling. When patients with cognitive deficits behave in a way that is inappropriate for the situation, or are slow to respond, healthcare workers must be careful not to view them as unmotivated, uncooperative, stubborn, or difficult. By altering the pattern of interaction with the patient, by restructuring the environment or the task, and by redesigning treatment goals, the rehabilitation of cognitively impaired patients remains an achievable goal. Cognitive deficits do not preclude learning and active participation in the rehabilitative process.

REFERENCES

1. Parkinson J: An Essay on the Shaking Palsy. Neely and Jones, London, 1817
2. Huber SJ, Paulson GW: The concept of subcortical dementia. Am J Psychiatry 142:1312, 1985
3. American Psychiatric Association: Diagnostic and statistical manual of mental disorders. 3rd Ed., Revised. American Psychiatric Association, Washington, DC, 1987
4. Albert ML, Feldman RG, Willis AL: The "subcortical dementia" of progressive supranuclear palsy. J Neurol Neurosurg Psychiatry 37:121, 1974
5. Steele JC, Richardson JC, Olszewski J: Progressive supranuclear palsy. Arch Neurol 10:333, 1964
6. Mayeux R, Stern Y: Intellectual dysfunction and dementia in Parkinson disease. p. 211. In Mayeux R, Rosen WG (eds): The Dementias. Raven Press, New York, 1983
7. Cummings JL, Benson DF: Subcortical dementia: Review of an emerging concept. Neurol Rev 41:874, 1984
8. Whitehouse PJ: The concept of subcortical and cortical dementia: Another look. Ann Neurol 19:1, 1986
9. Rajput AH, Offord K, Beard CM, Kurland LT: Epidemiological survey of dementia

in Parkinsonism and control population. p. 229. In Hassler RG, Christ JF (eds): Advances in Neurology. Vol. 40. Raven Press, New York, 1984

10. Mayeux MD, Stern Y, Rosen J, Benson DF: Is "subcortical dementia" a recognizable clinical entity? Ann Neurol 14:278, 1983

11. Mayeux R, Stern Y, Rosenstein R et al: An estimate of the prevalence of dementia in idiopathic Parkinson's disease. Arch Neurol 45:260, 1988

12. Ebmeir KP, Calder SA, Crawford JR: Clinical features predicting dementia in idiopathic Parkinson's disease: A follow-up study. Neurology 40:1222, 1990

13. Hietanen M, Teravainen H: The effect of age of disease onset on neuropsychological performance in Parkinson's disease. J Neurol Neurosurg Psychiatry 51:244, 1988

14. Sayetta RB: Rates of senile dementia—Alzheimer's type in the Baltimore longitudinal study. J Chron Dis 39:271, 1986

15. Oyebode JR, Barker WA, Blessed G et al: Cognitive functioning in Parkinson's disease: In relation to prevalence of dementia and psychiatric diagnosis. Br J Psychiatry 149:720, 1986

16. Mayeux R, Stern Y, Rosen J, Leventhal J: Depression, intellectual impairment, and Parkinson disease. Neurology 31:645, 1981

17. Caine, ED: Pseudodementia: Current concepts and future directions. Arch Gen Psychiatry 38:1359, 1981

18. Rabins PV: Psychopathology of Parkinson's disease. Comp Psychiatry 23:421, 1982

19. Sano M, Stern Y, Williams J et al: Coexisting dementia and depression in Parkinson's disease. Arch Neurol 46:1284, 1989

20. Taylor AE, Saint-Cyr JA, Lang AE, Kenny FT: Parkinson's Disease and depression: A critical re-evaluation. Brain 109:279, 1986

21. Starkstein SE, Berthier ML, Bolduc PL et al: Depression in patients with early versus late onset of Parkinson's disease. Neurology 39:1441, 1989

22. Mayberg HS, Starkstein SE, Sadzot B et al: Selective hypometabolism in the inferior frontal lobe in depressed patients with Parkinson's disease. Ann Neurol 28:57, 1990

23. Brown RG, MacCarthy B, Gotham AM et al: Depression and disability in Parkinson's disease: A follow-up of 132 cases. Psychol Med 18:49, 1988

24. Sagar JH, Cohen NH, Sullivan EV et al: Remote memory function in Alzheimer's disease and Parkinson's disease. Brain 111:185, 1988

25. El-Awar M, Becker JT, Hammond KM et al: Learning deficits in Parkinson's disease: Comparison with Alzheimer's disease and normal aging. Arch Neurol 44:180, 1987

26. Lees AJ, Smith E: Cognitive deficits in the early stages of Parkinson's disease. Brain 106:257, 1983

27. Milner B: Effects of different brain lesions on card sorting: The role of the frontal lobes. Arch Neurol 9:90, 1963

28. Levin BE, Llabre MM, Weiner WJ: Cognitive impairments associated with early Parkinson's disease. Neurology 39:557, 1989

29. Kimura D, Hahn A, Barnett HJM: Attentional and perseverative impairment in two cases of familial fatal Parkinsonism with cortical sparing. Can J Neurol Sci 14:597, 1987

30. Pirozzolo FJ, Hansch EC, Mortimer JA et al: Dementia in Parkinson's disease: A neuropsychological analysis. Brain Cogn 1:71, 1982

31. Hovestadt A, De Jong GJ, Meerwaldt JD: Visuospatial impairment in Parkinson's disease: Does it exist? J Neurol Neurosurg Psychiatry 50:1560, 1987

32. Spinnler H, Della Sala S: Visuo-spatial impairment in Parkinson's disease. Does it exist? J Neurol Neurosurg Psychiatry 50:1560, 1987

33. Brown RG, Marsden CD: Visuospatial functionin Parkinson's disease. Brain 109:987, 1986

34. Della Sala S, Di Lorenzo G, Giordano A, Spinnler H: Is there a specific visuo-spatial impairment in Parkinsonians? J Neurol Neurosurg Psychiatry 49:1258, 1986
35. Boller F, Passafiume D, Keefe NC et al: Visuospatial impairment in Parkinson's disease. Arch Neurol 41:485, 1984
36. Hovestadt A, De Jong GJ, Meerwaldt JD: Spatial disorientation as an early symptom of Parkinson's disease. Neurology 37:485, 1987
37. Hovestadt A, De Jong GJ, Meerwaldt JD: Spatial disorientation in Parkinson's disease: No effect of levodopa substitution therapy. Neurology 38:1802, 1988
38. Huber SJ, Shuttleworth EC, Freidenberg DL: Neuropsychological differences between the dementias of Alzheimer's and Parkinson's diseases. Arch Neurol 46:1287, 1989
39. Damasio AR: Language and the basal ganglia. Trends Neurosci 6:442, 1983
40. Streifler M, Hofman S: Disorders of verbal expression in Parkinsonism. p. 385. In Hassler RG, Christ JF (eds): Advances in Neurology. Vol. 40. Raven Press, New York, 1984
41. Darkins AW, Fromkin VA, Benson DF: A characterization of the prosodic loss in Parkinson's disease. Brain Lang 34:315, 1988
42. Matison R, Mayeux R, Rosen J, Fahn S: "Tip-of-the-tongue" phenomenon in Parkinson disease. Neurology 32:567, 1982
43. Kaplan E, Goodglass, H, Weintraub S: Boston Naming Test. Philadelphia, Lea & Febiger, 1983.
44. Beatty, WW, Monson N: Lexical Processing in Parkinson's disease and Multiple Sclerosis. J Ger Psychiatry Neurol 2:145, 1989
45. Mayeux R, Stern Y, Sano M et al: Clinical and biochemical correlates of bradyphrenia in Parkinson's disease. Neurology 37:1130, 1987
46. Pillon B, Dubois B, Bonnet AM et al: Cognitive slowing in Parkinson's disease fails to respond to levodopa treatment: The 15-objects test. Neurology 39:762, 1989
47. Evarts EV, Teravainen H, Calne DB: Reaction time in Parkinsons' disease. Brain 104:167, 1981
48. Dubois B, Pillon B, Legault F: Slowing of cognitive processing in progressive supranuclear palsy: A comparison with Parkinson's disease. Arch Neurol 45:1194, 1988
49. Posner MI: Orienting of attention. Q J Exp Psychol 32:3, 1980
50. Rafal RD, Posner MI, Walker JA, Freidrich FJ: Cognition and the basal ganglia: Separating mental and motor components of performance in Parkinson's disease. Brain 107:1083, 1984
51. Wright MJ, Burns RJ, Geffen GM, Geffen LB: Covert orientation of visual attention in Parkinson's disease: An impairment in the maintenance of attention. Neuropsychologia 28:151, 1990
52. Goodrich S, Henderson L, Kennard C: On the existence of an attention-demanding process peculiar to simple reaction time: Converging evidence from Parkinson's disease. Cogn Neuropsychol 6:309, 1989
53. Brown RG, Marsden CD: Internal versus external cues and the control of attention in Parkinson's disease. Brain 111:323, 1988
54. Norman DA, Shallice T: Attention to action: Willed and automatic control of behaviour. University of California CHIP Report 99, 1980
55. Baddeley A: Working Memory. Oxford University Press, Oxford, 1986
56. Dubinsky RM, Gray C, Husted D et al: Driving in Parkinsons' disease. Neurology 41:517, 1991

7 | The Role of Physical Therapy Intervention

George I. Turnbull

According to Schenkman and Butler,[1] there are three fundamental issues to consider when contemplating treatment for the patient with Parkinson's disease (PD). The first is to determine symptoms caused by the disease in a direct sense. Examples would be rigidity, tremor, and bradykinesia. The second issue pertains to those symptoms that appear secondarily to the actual disease process. These would include the fixed skeletal kyphosis and the habitual, flexed posture of the elbows, hips, and knees seen in patients in the later stages of the disease. A third group of symptoms are caused by the composite effect of the disturbances of both the central nervous system and the musculoskeletal system, and which involve such functional competencies as gait, balance, and transitional movements from one position to another (transfers). Schenkman and Butler are of the opinion that little can be done for those symptoms that result directly from the disease process itself, but that the second group, which they have referred to as the "musculoskeletal" or "non-nervous system" symptoms, may well be amenable to preventive strategies or even remediation by the physical therapist. By tackling the second group, the third or composite group of symptoms will also be improved to some extent. This basis for clinical decision making is extremely sound, and could form a useful starting point when considering how to proceed in developing programs for patients with PD.

While conceding that it is highly unlikely that physical therapy can influence the disease process of PD, there are indications that some of the more direct clinical symptoms of the disease can be improved, albeit for extremely short periods, by the use of physical therapy techniques that have been discovered accidently or through reasoning that may appear obscure. For example, a recent study by Bagley et al.[2] showed that visual cues improved certain spatial gait parameters in a group of PD patients, and that when the cues were removed there was a degree of carryover of that improvement. This is an interesting finding. The visual cues, which were triangular sections of brightly colored bristol board displayed at predetermined distances along a transduced walkway, improved the spatial parameters of the gait pattern during the walks in which the cues were introduced and for the walk that followed. This carryover effect demonstrates that the introduction of these cues resulted in an effect after they were removed. Although it is highly unlikely that these effects are of anything but an extremely short term nature, they can still be useful to the physical therapist and the patient in solving immediate problems of function. Furthermore, the research of Stelmach and Phillips, presented in this book, supports the idea that the learning of motor strategies can occur in PD patients, thus improving their performance. This therefore begs the question of whether the sufficiently frequent repetition of a short-term gain would result in more permanent improvements of function. However, for this hypothesis to stand any chance of being proven true, motor-learning characteristics would have to be considered and implemented. This idea sounds fairly simple, but from a practical viewpoint it is extremely difficult. Concepts such as motivation, compliance, repetition, accurate feedback, and task analysis are readily achievable when considering the young athlete. However, when these principles are applied to the treatment of a disorder such as PD, their application is a complicated and challenging task. As a result, and as previously mentioned in the introduction of this book, it is likely that physical therapists may be forced to deviate from the traditional model of physical therapy in order to overcome these problems, so that management of the PD patient can be made more effective, relevant, and helpful. The application of motor-learning principles is not a new concept in the area of neurologic rehabilitation. The motor-relearning program advocated by Carr and Shepherd[3] and the conductive education model of Cotton and Kinsman[4] both adhere to realistic learning models in the psychomotor domain in the treatment of stroke, while Kinsman[5] has also applied the Petö principles in the treatment of PD.

Before proposing a model of care that may be applied to the management of the PD patient, it would seem appropriate to review the role of the physical therapist as it has evolved over the years. This will permit the identification of key elements of management that should be included in such a model.

Physical therapy of the PD patient can be subdivided into five basic categories:

1. Assessment of function and the stage of the disease
2. Prevention of secondary sequelae
3. The improvement of motor competencies
4. The education and advice of patients and caregivers
5. The treatment of later-stage complications

ASSESSMENT OF FUNCTION AND THE STAGE OF THE DISEASE

The assessment of the person with PD is a difficult process because of the many systems involved in the disease and the variety of ways in which the disease can present and affect its victims. Margaret Sharpe has provided a comprehensive review of the assessment process in Chapter 8 of this book. There have been a number of proposals about how assessment could be achieved in a manner that is reliable, valid, and helpful in determining the symptoms of PD in the individual patient and their magnitude, and in monitoring functional deterioration over time. The Hoehn and Yahr staging scale[6] attempted to categorize patients according to their level of disability, and Schwab[6a] had the objective of classifying the progression of the disease. Webster[7] advocated the scoring of various features associated with PD on a 0 (no involvement) to 3 (severe impairment) scale whose results could be summed to provide an expression of disability level. Recently, Melnick[8] proposed the use of a modification of Webster's system, while Franklyn[9] has suggested a method of evaluating functional activities such as stair climbing, rolling, transfers, dexterity, gait, posture, and rising from the floor. This latter assessment format was compiled in Great Britain by the Working Party of Physiotherapists and the Parkinson's Disease Society. Kinsman[10] has used a standardized video assessment system that records the undertaking of specific competencies which are later scored by two or more clinicians using a variation of the scale proposed by Webster.[7] In addition to enhancing reliability, the videotape provides a permanent record of the patient's performance that is useful in identifying trends of deterioration much more vividly than written reports. This is an important feature because early identification of a failing competency is enhanced, thus leading to the potential for immediate implementation of a remedial program. In attempts to gain a comprehensive profile of the condition of the patient, some workers have combined a number of systems under the heading of the Unified Parkinson's Disease Rating Scale.[11] This process permits the patient to be scored under the categories of Mentation, Behavior and Mood; Activities of Daily Living; Motor Examination; Complications of Therapy (which considers such phenomena as dyskinesias and the "on-off" syndrome); a modified Hoehn and Yahr Staging Scale; and the Schwab and England Activities of Daily Living Scale. Although extremely comprehensive, this system is complex and time consuming, and is less than convenient for the patient. However, in certain circumstances, such as in the evaluation of radical new approaches to the treatment of PD, this is an appropriate option. However, for regular physical therapy assessment, this procedure is probably too cumbersome.

Irrespective of the technique used, there are three objectives of the assessment process. The first is to identify specific symptoms so that individualized treatment can be implemented. Although PD affects people in a manner that is somewhat predictable, the focus and severity of the symptoms will vary from one patient to another. The identification of the way in which the disease is affecting each individual, and the functional loss that results, have to be carefully identified before effective, targeted management can occur.

The second objective of assessment is to monitor function so that the insidious onset of a symptom can be detected and treated rapidly. The types of symptoms experienced by the PD patient are to some extent predictable, and regular monitoring for the appearance of these symptoms is therefore, not necessarily an arduous task.

The third objective may appear to be somewhat abstract but is nonetheless important. There is a need to form a database that will permit those working with PD patients to justify, through research, the validity of intervention. This is a most important function. In addition to the urgent need in physical therapy to justify the efficacy of the management techniques that are used, research can greatly influence whether or not patients with certain diseases receive appropriate treatment. For example, in the United States, insurance agencies frequently dictate the length of treatment a given patient can receive. The time frames developed by these companies have been derived from the "cure" philosophy mentioned earlier in this book. However, these agencies should be convinced that this paradigm is totally unsuitable in the treatment of PD and many other conditions. In Canada and the United Kingdom, where there is a more socialized approach to healthcare, similar problems exist but for different reasons. In those countries, priority is given to patients with acute disorders, a category into which the person with PD does not fit. Physical therapy for the PD patient is therefore also restricted in these systems of healthcare delivery. The only way that change can be convincingly brought about for the benefit of the PD patient is to generate sound research to substantiate claims that physical therapy is helpful and cost efficient in the management of PD. In order for this to be done on the magnitude needed to create the desired change, the development of a standardized database is vital. Perhaps it would be useful for physical therapists to adopt a common assessment format for PD that would result in widespread collaboration relating to the profile of the progression of the disease and the evaluation of a number of physical therapy interventions.

PREVENTION OF SECONDARY SEQUELAE

The gradual deterioration of function in the PD patient is well known. Recent advances in drug therapy will provide the patient with a longer functional expectancy than at any time in the past. However, these medications will eventually become ineffective or unpredictable and the patient will become increasingly disabled. The physical therapist, however, has the tools to do much to slow the inevitable onset of these complications. One such complication, often not identified, is a gradual deterioration in the patient's level of conditioning. As society becomes more aware of lifestyle and maintaining optimum levels of conditioning, a great deal is written and practiced about fitness, particularly among older members of society. The underlying philosophy is that maintaining optimal muscle strength, joint flexibility, cardiovascular fitness, and balance will lead to a fuller lifestyle than if these objectives are not pursued. For example, participation in programs of modified aerobics among seniors probably results in fewer accidental falls.[12] The sedentary lifestyle of elderly persons is often cited as a possible cause of some age-related events, such as idiopathic gait disorder of the elderly.[13] Thus, it would appear to be sensible for older people to exercise in order to enhance their lifestyle by ensuring that the cardiovascular, musculoskeletal, and neuromuscular systems are functioning at an optimal level. This trend among the general population is also entirely applicable to the person with PD, and indeed to all people with movement disorders. The detrimental effects of deconditioning have been proposed as difficult variables to treat following stroke, and may affect the outcome of the rehabilitation process in general.[3,14] As a result, it makes a great deal of sense for all people who have been diagnosed as having PD to undertake a general conditioning program upon diagnosis of the disorder, so that thay can maintain an optimal level of physical function. According to King, in Chapter 2 of this book, there is a 7-year window of opportunity from initial diagnosis to the time when medications begin to become ineffective. It is proposed that this 7-year period could be used to optimize the physical condition of the patient before the more traditional symptoms of PD become apparent.

When considering the typical secondary complications of PD, the increasing flexion deformities or the loss of rotation associated with such functional movements as gait are easily recognized. However, the phenomenon of learned non-use of normal motor function probably also occurs. Learned non-use has been cited as a factor that needs to be addressed in the rehabilitation of patients with disorders of the central nervous system[15] and stroke.[16] The use of this term means that the individual with PD becomes less able to generate a movement, and upon repeated failure stops trying to produce it. As a result, the movement-generated sensory feedback associated with a normal function is "forgotten," and the ability to detect when a movement is incorrect is lost. The disappearance of a kinesthetic memory specific to a given movement leaves the patient with an inability to produce efficient functional movements on demand. Instead, the patient perceives the abnormal movement pattern as "correct." The cliche of "use it or lose it" becomes the case. Therefore, any exercise program should also allow the patient with early PD the opportunity to rehearse and, therefore, retain normal functional movements, thus slowing the functional deterioration that accompanies the disease.

With regard to the more commonly recognized complications that arise from PD, Harrison[17] has drawn attention to the increasing postural discrepancies that occur over time. Other authors also stress the need to expose the PD patient to a program that will minimize the overall flexion that occurs in the spine, shoulders, elbows, hips, and knees.[18] Carr and Shepherd[19] have cited orofacial dysfunction and chest problems as being worthy of attention from a preventive viewpoint. Normal gait and appropriate postural awareness are mentioned by Franklyn[9] as targets of early care, while Kinnear[20] stresses the minimizing of secondary muscle weakness and joint stiffness, improvement of the depth of respiration, and the monitoring and correction of postural and gait discrepancies. In addition to the slow progression of clinical symptoms of rigidity, bradykinesia, and tremor, the PD patient's facial musculature, speech, and initiation of movement can also be expected to become problems that will interfere with function. The inclusion of preventive measures and/or the teaching of compensatory strategies to slow the progression of these predictable complications and their impact on function would also be a significant part of an early intervention program.

THE IMPROVEMENT OF MOTOR COMPETENCIES

In an attempt to organize the presentation of information to the reader, there is a tendency to put material into categories. In describing the care of the PD patient, there are some real dangers in doing this because the categories are not mutually exclusive entities. This is important for the reader to recognize. The PD patient does not, one day, appear in the physical therapy department and suddenly get transferred from a preventive to a remedial program. The transition is extremely gradual, and may take place over an extended period. I am reminded of the post-meniscectomy classes for knee rehabilitation of some 20 years ago. A patient could be a member of the non-weight-bearing group on a Monday, engaging in one hundred and one ways to perform static quadriceps contractions, and by Wednesday of the same week be promoted to the hustle and bustle of the partial-weight-bearing group. This example again is characteristic of the "cure" model. In the case of the PD patient, the ratio of time spent in preventive procedures to time spent in improving failing function will alter gradually as the condition of the patient deteriorates. However, in this section of the discussion, in which the improvement of motor competencies is considered, it is likely that elements of this component may also be a part of the preventive component of management previously addressed, and vice versa.

In addition to bradykinesia, rigidity, and tremor, the symptoms classically associated with PD, patients also develop a number of additional motor symptoms which are only now beginning to be understood. The PD patient suffers from a defect in motor planning,[21] and there is a deficiency in movement initiation and preparation.[8] These phenomena are addressed by Stelmach and Phillips in this book. It is likely that these decrements cause such symptoms as losing movement fluency when distracted, loss of normal automatic movements such as arm swing during gait, and freezing as obstacles are encountered. Isaacs (personal communication, 1987) studied the effects of PD patients being confronted with a doorframe built over a walkway designed to measure gait kinematics, and found that the gait pattern became tentative with increased festination as the patient approached the frame, despite the absence of a door in the frame. This is not an easy phenomenon to appreciate, but most PD patients will complain bitterly about this embarrassing event when they lose all ability to maintain movement (akinesia). For people who are normal—and physical therapists may boldly put themselves in this category—it is difficult to even remotely conceptualize these symptoms from an everyday functional viewpoint. Discussing them from a pathophysiologic perspective is helpful in understanding the mechanism of the disorder, but reveals little about its functional impact.

Physical therapists can gain a lot from listening carefully to the PD "folklore," comprising anecdotes about how patients cope under difficult circumstances. Terry Thomas, the British comedian and a great chocolate lover, was reputed to have candies hidden in various parts of his home so that, when he "froze" at a doorway, he could divert his thought processes to the chocolate on the other side of the door and, by doing this, unstick himself and so complete his journey into the room. This would tend to imply some form of compensation involving motivation and movement. Parkinson's disease patients will also tell of the value of carrying objects such as rocks or crushed paper in their pockets so that they may provide themselves with visual cues to step over should freezing occur. This phenomenon of visual cueing was studied by Bagley et al.[2] and found to be helpful in improving gait.

I recall having a conversation one evening with the vice president of the Halifax branch of the Parkinson's Disease Foundation. He was a man about 45 years old and had recently been diagnosed as having PD. He suddenly stopped talking in mid-sentence and told me how lucky I was. When I asked why, he told me how nice it must be to be able to stand up straight without thinking about it. Only by diverting his attention toward this previously automatic motor act was he able to stand straight. As we talked, his attention was focussed on the conversation, resulting in the gradual adoption of a flexed posture. I remember being struck forcefully by his comments and by the fact that we take our automatic movements so much for granted and, therefore, have a limited appreciation of the effect of this disease on the motor system despite all our knowledge. Another example of the bizarre movement disorder from which PD patients suffer was illustrated when I happened to observe a PD patient attempt several times to stand up from a sitting position. The person grasped the arms of a chair and made a few unsuccessful attempts to stand. This was followed by a period of complete immobility—an event made more dramatic by the fixed expression on his face. A passing physical therapist then told the man to move his head upward and forward when he was rising and, like magic to the untrained eye, he rose graciously to his feet and commenced walking. He had lost the skill of standing up. Initially, he had attempted to rise by extending his legs, but omitted all the preparatory work such as shifting his weight forward and placing his feet in the correct position under his center of mass. He did not lean forward at the waist to shift his center of mass forward. This observation can probably be explained by the work of Denny-Brown,[22] who described the role of the basal ganglia in producing an activating set that prepares the postural background so that a motor response appropriate to the environment can take place. This deficiency explains the difficulties of PD patients in initiating, changing, or halting movements as demanded by environmental variables. By simple coaching, the passing physical therapist had provided the patient described above with cognitive strategies related to these automatic adjustments, and he had succeeded perfectly well when he implemented them. The tragedy of this situation is that this positive effect is of short duration and is quickly extinguished.

The physical therapist is, therefore, faced with the treatment of a number of motor problems. Included in this list are bradykinesia, akinesia, rigidity, loss of voluntary initiation, alteration, or cessation of movement, and loss of normal automatic motor acts such as arm swing and postural control. These symptoms will involve the patient's skeletal muscles as well as those of facial expression, speech, chewing, and swallowing, and bring with them a host of functional decrements relating to activities of daily living. However, there are a number of movement strategies available to the physical therapist which appear to assist the quality of movement of which the patient is capable. Rotational movements of the extremities and spine appear to reduce rigidity, albeit for short periods.[23] Active-assisted exercises (pumping up or rhythmic intention), in which the physical therapist assists the patient and gradually withdraws assistance as the patient responds by developing a "head of steam," can for a short period overcome problems related to the initiation of movement.[19] This becomes functionally viable if the movement is performed in functional patterns such as those proposed by Knott and Voss.[24] These particular techniques, however, should be modified, because "freeing" the patient and not strengthening is the objective. Therefore, the use of resistance and the application of techniques of emphasis appear to be inappropriate. Relaxation procedures have also been found to be of some use, as have gentle rocking techniques,[23] particularly when this rocking incorporates counter-rotation between the shoulder girdle and the pelvis. Cueing the patient in a rhythmic manner also has been reported to be of help, using dance,[25] counting, and visual cues.[26] Exaggerated movement such as goose stepping over obstacles[18] and facilitating arm swing by mechanically moving the patient at the hips or shoulders[27] also seems to be associated with functional gains over the short term.

As has been previously noted and often repeated, these techniques, which most clinicians who have worked with PD patients will recognize, do something, but the effect is not sustained. This, however, is not an uncommon feature when dealing with the patient suffering from neurologic dysfunction. In the treatment of the stroke patient, it is possible to reduce spasticity and achieve more normal movement during the course of a treatment session. The difficulty is in maintaining those gains so that they may be integrated into the habitual patterns of movement of the patient, thus improving function. Perhaps it would be fruitful to consider how people learn new movement skills and incorporate these principles into management programs for the patient with PD. This is not an unreasonable suggestion considering the knowledge that short-term improvements can be achieved in PD, and that patients with the disease appear capable of improving performance through learning. The assumption, therefore, is that more permanent gains may be possible if the patient "learns" the desired maneuver, and that as function begins to deteriorate, early detection can salvage the deteriorating functional activity by planned practice of that activity. A major diversion of this approach from the domain of psychomotor learning is that many of the tasks that have to be learned therapeutically are not regarded as skills. Activities of daily living are not usually associated with formal learning processes, but when it is considered that all of us, at some stage of our lives, were taught to tie our shoelaces, dress, and even stand up, the application of psychomotor learning theory does make some sense. What, therefore, are the key variables that are most likely to permit these short-term gains in the PD patient to become more permanent, and how can they be realistically implemented into an overall management model? In attempts to answer this question, it is necessary to consider some principles of learning in the psychomotor domain.

Learning can be defined as a change in the internal state of the individual that is inferred from a relatively permanent improvement in performance and as a result of practice.[28] Although learning is not directly observable, it can be implied from behavior or performance.[28] Learning can occur in the cognitive domain, which is usually associated with intellectual activities, the affective domain, which pertains to emotional control and moral judgements, and the psychomotor domain, which deals with the acquisition of perceptual or motor skills.[28] All three learning domains are interdependent upon each other, but for descriptive purposes they are often treated separately. The psychomotor domain, because of its relevance to movement-related activities, is of direct relevance to the physical therapist, and may hold the answers to the questions posed above.[29]

According to Fitts,[30] psychomotor learning occurs in three phases. The first phase is the cognitive phase, during which the learner acquires the principles of the task to be accomplished. In the physical therapy department, this is usually done by explaining to the patient what is required, highlighting key features to which the patient must attend. It should, however, be pointed out that the physical therapist may neglect this phase of the motor-learning process. It may seem redundant to explain such a fundamental skill as standing up from a chair. However, it was exactly this explanation that helped the patient discussed earlier. As a result, it would probably be wise for the physical therapist to pay more attention to key parts of the movement, particularly those that are most likely to be performed incorrectly. The cognitive phase usually lasts for only a short time, following which the learner progresses to the fixation phase.

The fixation phase of psychomotor learning is the component of skill acquisition in which the learner attempts to reduce the number of errors in performance of a skill, an objective achieved through repetition and the provision and utilization of feedback. It has been known for some time that repetition without feedback is ineffective.[31] It can be said that practice does not make perfect, it makes permanent. Therefore, repetition of a motor act performed incorrectly will lead to a habituation of errors that may later be difficult to rectify. Thus, accurate feedback to the learner is essential as the skill is rehearsed. There are two types of feedback. Knowledge of results (KR) is provided by externally generated information which permits the learner to determine the success of his or her performance through the accomplishment of a goal or recognition of the extent of failure to accomplish the goal. Knowledge of performance (KP) is generated by whether or not the movement pattern used in accomplishing a task was appropriate to the task.[32] Knowledge of performance is usually provided by a coach or knowledgeable observer initially until such time as the learner develops enough of a frame of reference to judge the quality of his or her own performance when undertaking the task. Both systems of feedback are vital to the efficient acquisition of a skill. It can be seen, therefore, that the physical therapist is a coach of movement during this phase of skill acquisition, and is a major supplier of feedback to the patient as the patient attempts to relearn a functional competency. As the degree of error declines and the performance of the target task becomes more efficient, the patient will be able to provide an autonomous measure of KP, and this is an important objective in psychomotor learning for the PD patient, particularly when the issue of learned non-use, described earlier, is considered.

Another consideration that must be addressed in the fixation phase of learning is the nature of the task to be learned. It is known that more complex tasks require different training strategies than simple tasks.[33] Given that the skills being acquired in the context of the PD patient are activities of daily living, the physical therapist will greatly enhance the acquisition of an activity if remedial measures are enacted as soon as errors become apparent. This means that only those components of the pattern of movement that are becoming deficient will need to be practiced and then reintegrated into the overall movement pattern. However, for this system to work, sensitive evaluation methods are essential, as is the opportunity for the physical therapist to intervene in a timely fashion. Two months on a waiting list will probably result in the patient deteriorating to a level at which the problem becomes irreversible. The construction of a program of management for the PD patient must therefore ensure the prompt association of intervention with the early detection of functional deterioration.

It can be seen that sufficiently frequent practice with feedback will be required before realistic motor learning can occur. It is probable that the learner would be expected to practice every day, and this daunting requirement presents a host of additional problems. Motivation and compliance are extremely difficult matters with which to deal. This is particularly true of the patient with PD, who may have difficulties with motivation. How then can these problems be addressed? It is known that the learner has to perceive a new skill as worth acquiring.[32] It is also known that locus of control affects the motivation to comply with health-related behaviors.[34,35] Persons who feel that they are not in control of their situation have been shown to be less motivated than those who perceive a measure of control over critical factors. This principle has been widely adopted in the business world. Consequently, it is important to provide the patient with a feeling of control over his or her destiny. This can be achieved, at least in part, by involving the patient and, if necessary, the caregiver, in the formulation of a management program. Sculpting the program around the wants, needs, and desires of the patient and listening to the patient's opinions about the content of the exercise program, will enable the patient to begin to feel a sense of ownership in the program, with a greater likelihood of taking more responsibility in complying with it. It is important for the physical therapist to present options to the patient, who should feel an integral part of the decisionmaking process. This is not a traditional role for the physical therapist, who in the past has tended to decide what is best for the patient. However, PD patients are not traditional patients, and a change of functioning on the part of the physical therapist may therefore be required. The adoption of this proposed change in role by the physical therapist ascribes a partnership role to the patient, rather than the role of a subordinate. The responsibility this generates will provide the patient with a vested interest in the patient's ongoing exercise program, and is therefore more likely to ensure greater motivation and compliance.

Another psychomotor learning concept that may be of considerable use to the PD patient is mental rehearsal. A number of researchers have shown that mental practice is beneficial to the performance of a well learned skill and to the acquisition of a new skill.[28] Mental practice is the cognitive rehearsal of a physical skill in the absence of overt physical practice.[28] The high jumper who stands while preparing to jump and mentally rehearses the perfect jump is likely to jump more efficiently than the athlete who does not do this. The concept is widely practiced in sophisticated sports competition. The basketball player will rehearse a foul shot before its execution, while a diver can mentally run through the necessary movement sequence before the dive takes place. Although it has never been the subject of a research study, the extrapolation of this concept to the PD population would seem to be productive unless the cognitive capabilities of the patient were diminished. Cognitively rehearsing a transfer from standing to sitting could, for example, improve the performance of the transfer. This may require that the patient be taught a cognitive strategy to rehearse before attempting to undertake the movement. Such an approach may have helped the functional ability of the patient described earlier, who was attempting to stand up from a sitting position.

After a variable period that depends heavily on the complexity of the task being acquired, the learner will enter the final stage of skill acquisition, the autonomous phase. In this phase, the skill can be executed in a highly efficient manner without the concentration demands of earlier stages of the learning process. The learner is able to divert more attention to other aspects of performance of the skill. The astute reader will recognize that this final phase is exactly what the PD patient loses: the ability to carry out automatic activities with minimal demands on attention. Nevertheless, this would seem to be a valid objective in the treatment of the PD patient, except that providing the environment for this level of acquisition to occur is a difficult proposition in the case of the PD patient.

Another feature of the autonomous phase of acquiring a skill is that even in professional athletes, the skill can begin to break down. This probably results from small errors in performance that appear and grow as they are repeated. These errors are usually associated with deteriorating efficiency in performing the skill, and require a return to earlier phases of skill acquisition for their eradication. This will probably happen regularly with the PD patient. As the disease progresses, movement errors will appear and result in a breakdown of performance. A critical element of the role of the physical therapist is to be able to detect these movement errors and intervene in a timely manner. This will call upon the abilities and knowledge of the physical therapist for analyzing the abnormal pattern of movement, detecting its discrepancy from the desired pattern, and instituting remedial steps to rebuild the movement pattern by drawing the patient's attention to the errors and proposing ways to correct the abnormality. This may necessitate a return to the cognitive phase of motor learning and then to the fixation phase with accentuated practice, initially with enhanced feedback. It will probably also require the application of some of the specialized physical therapy techniques described earlier.

In time, the patient will become incapable of ideal performance. When this occurs, the physical therapist may begin to divert attention to the teaching of motor patterns that can compensate for diminishing motor abilities, thus preserving function for as long as possible. Again, the application of techniques to reduce such symptoms as rigidity and defective initiation of movement may be required.

Any long-term management program in which attempts are made to improve functional movement will eventually have the objective of the relearning of functional psychomotor skills. The use of principles from the theory of motor learning would therefore seem to be an essential ingredient of such a program.

EDUCATION AND ADVICE OF PATIENTS AND CARE GIVERS

Parkinson's disease is a condition that can be considered obscure as far as its symptoms and clinical progression are concerned. Heart disease, in contrast, is well known because it is often dramatized and depicted in the media. On the contrary, PD is shrouded in mystery and lack of knowledge. Most people are unaware of its precise nature unless they have some direct experience of it. Consequently, there is a need to educate the PD patient and the patient's family or caregivers about what the disease entails, the medications involved, their side effects, what preventive steps can be taken to minimize complications, and how specific symptoms can best be managed. This problem can be solved in a number of ways, but it is probably most appropriate to allow PD patients and their families to find the solution most appropriate for themselves. This is consistent with the concept of self determination discussed earlier. Community based groups have been shown to be viable vehicles for this sort of activity, and stroke clubs, Huntington's Disease and PD Society chapters play an invaluable role in this regard in serving their constituents. It is also likely that a number of healthcare professionals would be involved in this type of activity. How then can the physical therapist contribute to these groups in a manner that will be beneficial to their members? The physical therapist has a lot to offer in teaching PD patients and their caregivers about movement in general, how PD affects normal movement, and what strategies might be attempted in solving functional problems. The identification of secondary side effects will probably enhance the patient's motivation to perform activities designed to slow the onset of these complications, and the caregivers can be taught basic techniques that will assist in the day-to-day care of the PD patient. Clearly, in order to achieve these goals, the physical therapist will need some kind of forum in which to identify the patients' and caregivers' needs and to then teach the necessary material when required. This could be done in a hospital or community-based program, but it could also be linked to the activities of PD self-help groups. They meet frequently, have access to their membership through newsletters and other means, and become adept at rounding up members. This may seem time-consuming for the physical therapist, but it need not be. The development of video technology as well as desktop publishing techniques and other computer generated information is now at a stage at which these technologies are usable and are not merely a fanciful academic's dream. By utilizing such learning aids, along with the more traditional approaches such as lectures and small group discussions, a great deal can be accomplished in an efficient yet effective manner. In Halifax, the Nova Scotia Chapter of the Parkinson's Foundation of Canada has already progressed to the level at which some of these concepts have been implemented. The techniques used will be discussed at the end of this chapter.

THE TREATMENT OF LATER-STAGE COMPLICATIONS

As the medications used in treating PD become less effective in improving the patient's condition, secondary complications are likely to increase in both magnitude and frequency. The "on-off" phenomenon, in which the patient is likely to suddenly develop full-blown symptoms of PD despite being relatively functional immediately before this; the deterioration in performance as the medications wear off, combined with significant improvement as the next dose takes effect; and the appearance of dyskinesias are all symptoms with which the patient may have to learn to cope. Similarly, as the symptoms of the disease become more pronounced, there will be greater percentages of time during which the patient suffers from disabling symptoms than there will be periods of functional capability. In these circumstances, the objective of physical therapy will be to teach the caregiver techniques that will result in small, very short-term gains, but which may prove to be sufficient to allow the patient to reach a functional goal such as getting out of bed or finishing a meal. Obviously the physical therapist will not be with a patient at all times, particularly if the patient has to transfer from a lying to a sitting position to be given medication through the night. Therefore, teaching some basic techniques to the caregiver is essential. The effects of these techniques may be short-lived, but they may well make a difference to the care of the patient. Another important role of the physical therapist is to teach the patient how to plan the activities of the day around the disabling symptoms of the disease. It is not unusual for the PD patient at this stage of the disease to be functional only for the middle hour out of every three. In the first hour the patient is essentially disabled while the medication is taking effect; during the second hour, however, the patient can function as a result of the medication. During the third hour, the medication is wearing off, and this is accompanied by increasing disability. Planning activities for the second hour therefore becomes a priority.

As mentioned by Fox in Chapter 2 of this book, it may be deemed necessary, in the later stages of PD, to admit the patient to the hospital for the evaluation of medication or even for a drug "holiday." At this time, it would seem appropriate for the patient to receive an "intensive" dose of physical therapy in an attempt to improve function. This would include the treatment of orofacial and lung dysfunction.

In the late stages of PD, the patient will probably be dependent. The caregiver can still be helped a great deal by being shown such maneuvers as efficient ways to change the position of the patient in bed and how to prevent pressure sores. This is a difficult time for the caregiver, and the support of the healthcare team is essential. Late-stage complications of the disease would be treated symptomatically as the need arises, although it would seem wise to continue with such important preventive measures as breathing exercises and skin care.

CONCLUSION

As previously proposed, the realistic role of the physical therapist in the treatment of PD is not a traditional role. The likelihood of physical therapy being provided effectively in a traditional environment such as a hospital physical therapy department is limited. From the previous discussion it would seem that the inclusion of the following principles in such a program would be fundamental to its success:

1. The early implementation of an exercise program to prevent deconditioning and other preventable complications at the time of diagnosis of PD.
2. The utilization of a meaningful and practical assessment procedure that is relatively short but will permit the identification of treatment priorities on an individual basis and allow the progress of the patient to be monitored on a regular basis.
3. The identification of deterioration and timely intervention to compensate for failing competency.
4. The opportunity for the patient to reacquire a failing competency and to learn compensatory motor strategies and/or consolidate short-term gains through structured programs that adhere to known principles of psychomotor learning.
5. The involvement of the patient and the patient's caregivers in decision making to improve motivation and compliance with any exercise program.
6. A forum to identify the needs of the patient and caregivers, and in which to then teach material about PD and its effect on functional movement.
7. The teaching of techniques to the caregiver that will result in small, short-term gains but which will permit the patient's immediate attainment of a given functional objective.

How can the physical therapist attain these lofty theoretical principles in a manner that is efficient from the perspective of both time and economics?

There are probably a number of ways in which these objectives could be reached, and the solution would be dictated by a number of variables. In Halifax, Nova Scotia, a group of physical therapists, including some students working under supervision, have attempted to provide a practical solution to this question in close cooperation with the Halifax–Dartmouth Chapter of the Parkinson Foundation of Canada. The program has been constructed on the theoretical basis described in this chapter. Since the completion of this preliminary work, which was developed over a period of some 6 years, a number of enquiries have been made from throughout Canada to request information about the program and its content. In addition, similar programs have been set up in St John's, Newfoundland, and Saint John, New Brunswick. As a result of this interest and the apparent helpfulness of the program, it was felt that it would be useful to publish some of the information that the program has generated and to make suggestions about how the program could be enhanced. It is not being proposed as a universal panacea because adjustments would have to be made in the light of such factors as the size of the population being served, the geographic location of the area in which the program would be implemented, the facilities available, the enthusiasm and commitment of the PD community, and the interest within the physical therapy community.

It was decided to call the program the "HELP" program, an acronym for Helpful Exercises for Living with Parkinson's, and it is designed to be a multidimensional approach to the problem of PD. The total program includes a booklet with exercises, suggestions to improve function and a worksheet designed to improve motivation and a compliance with the exercise program; an exercise videotape that runs on a home video system (VHS) and contains exercises to address the prevention of complications, specific problems, and cardiovascular fitness that the patient can do at home in conjunction with the videotape; a physical therapist, who will meet with patients on a regular basis and whose role is to assess function, monitor progress and, in consultation with the patient or caregiver, determine the specific emphasis of the program; and any group of people, such as friends, family, and workmates of the patient who want to join in the exercises. The last option is an attempt to improve motivation and compliance, and usually comprises a group made up of other members of the PD society who are present at its monthly meetings or at the weekly exercise sessions run by the physical therapist.

The Current Booklet:

The booklet currently being used in the HELP program was developed as a pilot project by students in the physical therapy program of the School of Physiotherapy at Dalhousie University, working under the supervision of and in close cooperation with members of the physical therapy community and the membership of the Halifax–Dartmouth Chapter of the Parkinson Foundation of Canada. Attempts were made to produce an appealing publication at low cost, and desktop publishing techniques using an Apple MacIntosh computer were therefore used. The booklet was designed to allow the physical therapist to suggest exercises to suit the needs of the patient. Upon assessment of the condition of the patient, the physical therapist provides the patient with suggestions and a rationale for the direction of treatment. After discussion, a program is established that allows the patient to do many of the exercises at home, thus ensuring their sufficient repetition. The exercises are taught to the patient, and the illustrations in the booklet are included to remind the patient of the exercise being described. A key feature is that the physical therapist must provide the

PARKINSON'S DISEASE EVALUATION FORM

(Circle Appropriate Score)

Bradykinesia of hands

0   No involvement

1   Detectable slowing of supination/pronation rate evidenced by beginning difficulty in handling tools; buttoning clothes; and with handwriting.

2   Moderate slowing of supination/pronation rate, one or both sides, evidenced by moderate impairment of hand function. Handwriting is greatly impaired, micrographia

3   Severe slowing of supination/pronation rate. Unable to write or button clothes. Marked difficulty in handling utensils

Rigidity

0   Undetectable

1   Detectable rigidity in neck and shoulders. Activation phenomenon is present. One or both arms show mild, negative, resting rigidity

2   Moderate rigidity in neck and shoulders. Resting rigidity is positive when patient not on meds.

3   Severe rigidity in neck and shoulders. Resting rigidity cannot be reversed by meds.

Posture

0   Normal posture. Head forward flexed less than 4 inches

1   Beginning poker spine. Head flexed forward up to 5 inches

2   Beginning arm flexion. Head flexed forward up to 6 inches. One or both arms flexed but still below waist

3   Onset of Simian posture. Head flexed forward more than 6 inches. Sharp flexion of hand, beginning interphalangeal extension. Beginning flexion of knees.

Upper Extremity Swing

0   Swings both arms well

1   One arm decreased in amount of swing

2   One arm fails to swing

3   Both arms fail to swing

Gait

0   Step length is between 18-30 inches. Turns effortlessly

1   Step length shortened to 12-18 inches. Foot/floor contact abnormalities in one side. Turn around slowing and takes several steps

2   Step length 6 to 12 inches. Foot/floor contact abnormalities on both sides

3   Onset of shuffling gait. Occasional stuttering gait with feet sticking to floor. Walks on toes. Turns very slowly

Tremor

0   No tremor
1   Less than 1 inch amplitude tremor observed in limbs or head at rest or in either hand while walking
2   Maximum tremor envelope fails to exceed 4 inches. Tremor is severe but not constant. Patient still has some control of hands
3   Tremor envelope exceeds 4 inches. Tremor is constant and severe. Writing and feeding are impossible

Face

0   Normal. Full animation. No stare
1   Detectable immobility. Mouth remains closed. Beginning features of anxiety or depression
2   Moderate immobility. Emotion shows at markedly increased threshold. Lips parted some of the time. Moderate features of anxiety or depression. Drooling may occur.
3   Frozen face. Mouth slightly open. Severe drooling may be present

Speech

0   Clear, loud, resonant, easily understood
1   Beginning of hoarseness with loss of inflection and resonance. Good volume. Still easily understood
2   Moderate hoarseness and weakness. Constant monotone, unvaried pitch, early dysarthria, hesitancy, stuttering, difficult to understand
3   Marked hoarseness and weakness. Very difficult to hear and understand

Self-care

0   No impairment
1   Still provides full self-care but rate of dressing definitely slowed. Able to live alone and still employable
2   Requires help in certain critical areas such as turning in bed, rising from chairs etc. Very slow in performing most activities but manages by taking time
3   Continuously disabled. Unable to dress, feed self or walk alone

Overall Disability (Sum of the scores from all categories):

1 - 9 Early stage	10 - 18 Moderate disability	19 - 27 Severe or advanced stage

Fig. 7-1. Parkinson's Disease Evaluation Form. (Modified from Webster,[7] with permission.)

specific feedback to which the patient must attend to ensure that the exercises are being undertaken correctly. Similarly, a caregiver can be instructed about the feedback that must be provided to the patient about the patient's performance. The suggested exercises are reviewed with the patient on a regular basis, perhaps every third or fourth month, and adjusted as necessary. In addition, the physical therapist checks the worksheet schedule to ensure that compliance is occurring. It is interesting to note that patients so far enrolled in the program are scrupulously honest about their adherence to it. Most of the exercises proposed in the book also form part of the regular exercise program conducted by the physical therapist on a weekly basis, therefore providing ample opportunity for the exercises to be monitored. Furthermore, the patient is regularly reminded not to perform the exercises in a way that could be considered harmful. To date there have been no instances of problems in this area.

The Exercise Videotape

An exercise videotape has also been made as part of the HELP program, and was designed to be copied and used by patients in their own homes, again using available technology to limit cost. As a result, a VHS format was used. The exercises overlap to some degree those in the booklet and those given by the physical therapist at the weekly exercise sessions. They are done to a musical accompaniment that was judiciously chosen in terms of its rhythm, the exercise being undertaken, and the age of the majority of the patients. The exercises on the videotape are done by members of the Halifax, Nova Scotia chapter of the Parkinson Foundation of Canada, and the exercise session is led by the chapter's physical therapist. The prevention of PD-related complications and maintenance of functional activities and cardiovascular fitness are the objectives of the videotape. The videotape can periodically be revised to ensure that patients do not become bored with this aspect of the package. Old tapes can be re-dubbed as a means of reducing the cost to the patient.

The Physical Therapist

The physical therapist is critical to the success of the HELP program. As a result, the person who fills this role must have a deep interest in PD as a condition, and in the welfare of the patients he or she encounters. In addition, the therapist must have a clear understanding of his or her role in this context. The actual time involved is not great. The physical therapist in Halifax runs a 1-hour exercise session each week for interested participants, and also attends the monthly meetings of the chapter, which is a commitment of about 3 hours. It is at these meetings that the consultations with the patients and caregivers occur, and this is done on a staggered basis so that each patient is seen once over a period of about 4 months. During consultations, the physical therapist meets with the patient and if necessary with a caregiver. An assessment using a modified version of the system proposed by Webster[7] (Fig. 7-1) is used, and management objectives are developed as a result of this assessment. A personalized program is formulated with the input of the patient and caregiver. The physical therapist also has the responsibility of organizing patient records and updating resource materials. Once the system has been established, these are not arduous tasks. In addition, from time to time and as necessary, the physical therapist communicates the patient's progress to the patient's family physician.

The Local Parkinson's Disease Society

It has been my experience that self-help groups like those in the HELP program are extremely productive and highly motivated. In Halifax, the PD group is well consolidated and has its own facility for meetings and exercise sessions. In addition to regular input from the physical therapist, the group arranges to hear guest speakers from the fields of speech therapy, neurology, psychology, pharmacology, and other areas of relevance. The membership is extremely well informed and the discussions that follow presentations are lively and productive. Experiences are shared to the benefit of all who attend. The membership socializes together and also takes time out to discuss hobbies and other lighter topics with guests. There is a sense of comradeship, and the meetings are particularly beneficial to the patients' caregivers because they soon realize that they are not alone in their plight. This type of support is absolutely essential. Fundraising to promote research in the area of PD is also undertaken, and this often provides the membership with a sense of purpose and belonging. This forum is ideal for enhancing the nontraditional role of the physical therapist, and the environment is conducive to ensuring motivation and perseverance.

The content of the booklet is presented in the Appendix to this chapter for the consideration of members of the physical therapy community who are seeking solutions to the problem of dealing with PD patients.

REFERENCES

1. Schenkman M, Butler RB: A model for multisystem evaluation treatment of individuals with Parkinson's disease. Phys Ther 69:932, 1989
2. Bagley S, Kelly B, Tunnicliffe N et al: The effect of visual cues on the gait of independently mobile Parkinson's patients. Physiotherapy 77:415, 1991
3. Carr JH, Shepherd R: A Motor Relearning Programme for Stroke. Aspen, Rockville, Maryland, 1983
4. Cotton E, Kinsman R: Conductive Education for Adult Hemiplegia. Churchill Livingstone, Edinburgh, 1983
5. Kinsman R: Conductive education for the patient with Parkinson's disease. Physiotherapy 72:385, 1986

6. Hoehn MM, Yahr MD: Parkinsonism: onset, progression and mortality. Neurology 17:427, 1967

6a. Schwab RS: Progression and prognosis in Parkinson's disease. J Nerve Ment Dis 130:556, 1967

7. Webster D: Critical analysis of disability in Parkinson's disease. Mod Treat 5:257, 1968

8. Melnick ME: Basal ganglia disorders. Metabolic, hereditary and genetic disorders in adults. In Umphred, D (ed): Neurological Rehabilitation. C.V. Mosby, St. Louis, 1991

9. Franklyn S: An introduction to physiotherapy for Parkinson's disease. Physiotherapy 72:379, 1986

10. Kinsman R: Video assessment of the Parkinson patient. Physiotherapy 72:386, 1986b

11. Fine A, Fisk J, Heffernan L et al: Clinical trial of human fetal neural transplantation for therapy of Parkinson's disease. Unpublished Project Proposal, Dalhousie University, Halifax, Nova Scotia, 1991

12. Hogan DB, Wall JC, Beresford P et al: The effects of an exercise program on parameters of balance and gait in the elderly. In preparation, 1991

13. Wall JC, Hogan DB, Turnbull GI, Fox RA: The kinematics of idiopathic gait disorder of the elderly: a comparison with healthy young and elderly females. Scand J Rehab Med 23:159, 1991

14. Bach-y-Rita P: Recovery of Function: Theoretical Considerations for Brain Injury Rehabilitation. Hans Huber, Bern, 1981

15. Moore J: Neuroanatomical considerations relating to recovery of function following brain injury. In Bach-y-Rita, P (ed): Recovery of Function: Theoretical Considerations for Brain Injury Rehabilitation. Hans Huber, Bern, 1981

16. Turnbull GI: Motor learning theory. In Banks M (ed): International Perspectives in Physical Therapy—2. Stroke Churchill Livingstone, Edinburgh, 1986

17. Harrison MA: Parkinsonism—Physiotherapy. In Downie PA (ed): Cash's Textbook of Neurology for Physiotherapists. Faber and Faber, London, 1982

18. Cailliet R: Rehabilitation in parkinsonism. In Licht S (ed): Rehabilitation and Medicine. Licht, New Haven, Connecticut, 1968

19. Carr JH, Shepherd R: Physiotherapy in Disorders of the Brain. Henemann, London, 1980

20. Kinnear E: Long term management of Parkinson's disease. Physiotherapy 72:340, 1986

21. Chan CWY: Could Parkinsonian akinesia be attributable to a disturbance in the motor preparatory process? Brain Res 386:183, 1986

22. Denny-Brown D: The Basal Gangli and their Relation to Disorders of Movement. Liverpool University Press, Liverpool, 1962

23. Goff B: The application of recent advances in neurophysiology to Miss M. Rood's concept of neuromuscular facilitation. Physiotherapy 58:409, 1972

24. Knott M, Voss DE: Proprioceptive Neuromuscular Facilitation. Patterns and Techniques. Harper & Row, New York, 1968

25. Ball JM: Demonstration of the traditional approach in the treatment of a patient with Parkinsonism. Am J Phys Med 46:1034, 1967

26. Dunne JW, Hankey GJ, Edis RH: Parkinsonism: upturned walking stick as an aid to locomotion. Arch Phys Med Rehabil 68:380, 1987

27. McNiven DR: Rotational improvement of movement in the Parkinsonian patient. Physiotherapy 72:381, 1986

28. Magill RA: Motor Learning. Concepts and Applications. Brown, Dubuque, Iowa, 1980

29. Turnbull GI: Some learning theory implications in neurological physiotherapy. Physiotherapy 68:38, 1982
30. Fitts PM: Perceptual-motor skill learning. In Melton, AW (ed): Categories of Human Learning. Academic Press, New York, 1964
31. Trowbridge MH, Cason H: An experimental study of Thorndike's theory of learning. J Gen Psychol 7:245, 1932
32. Schmidt RA: Motor Control and Learning. A Behavioral Emphasis. Human Kinetics Publishers, Champaign, Illinois, 1982
33. Holding DH: Human Skills. John Wiley & Sons, New York, 1981
34. Steffy RA, Meichenbaum D, Best JA: Aversive and cognitive factors in the modification of smoking behavior. Behav Res Ther 8:115, 1970
35. Wallston BS, Wallston KA: Locus of control and health: a review of the literature. Health Ed Monogr 6:107, 1978

APPENDIX 7-1

"HELP" for Living with Parkinson's. A Program Designed for Persons with Parkinson's Disease and Their Families

TABLE OF CONTENTS

PD FACTS

In 1817 James Parkinson described a disease he called the **"shaking palsy"**
Later this became known as **Parkinson's Disease (PD)**

    PD is one of the **most common** neurologic disorders of the elderly, second only to stroke

    PD affects **1 in every 1,000 people** (considering the whole population)

    If we all lived long enough, **everyone** would develop **PD**

    It is **not known** why some people develop **PD**

    PD occurs **equally** in both sexes

    Life expectancy for people with **PD** is **increasing** because of advanced treatment techniques such as medications

    PD, like no other neurologic disorder, **has been helped** by the development of new medications

    Exercise can help **slow down** the appearance of complications from the disease and so preserve optimal function

    The best results achieved from an exercise treatment program occur if the program is started **early,** at the time of diagnosis

INTRODUCTION

This program is especially designed to assist the person with **PD.**

Purpose

This program is being offered to you to

1. Help you delay the onset of complications from **PD**
2. Teach you more about the disease and how it affects movement
3. Find ways to assist you to deal with your specific concerns
4. Improve your overall fitness

The Total Program Includes

1. **This booklet**—exercises, helpful hints, recording system, and more
2. **An exercise videotape**—exercises for specific problems, for preventing complications, and for fitness
3. **A physical therapist** who will help you develop and monitor the program
4. **Any group of people**—friends, family and workmates—who want to join in

THIS PROGRAM IS ONLY A MECHANISM TO HELP YOU **HELP YOURSELF.**

YOU ARE THE ONE WHO HAS TO BE RESPONSIBLE FOR MAKING IT WORK.

BENEFITS OF AN EXERCISE PROGRAM

Exercise is essential. An exercise program will **slow down** the appearance of complications from *PD* and improve your general **fitness** level.

PD affects people in **different ways** so a good exercise program should be specific for each person:

1. It will concentrate on areas that are of most concern to you
2. It will improve your quality of life
3. It will help you do things on your own for as long as possible

The fitness component of the exercise program:

1. Will help you stay in better shape both physically and mentally
2. Will help you be better able to deal with activities in your daily life and problems which may occur as a result of *PD*

Routine Work Sheet

This will help you REMEMBER your program and it should, we hope, give you more **incentive** to be faithful to the program (which is something we all need at times). Incentive can also be improved if you arrange to exercise with your friends.

THE ROLE OF PHYSICAL THERAPY

A physical therapist is there to offer you advice and assistance that can help you in your activities of every day living. In particular, the physical therapist will be interested in how you move and will assess your movement performance in various tasks and suggest ways to help you.

She/he can help you by formulating an individualized exercise program, which will be designed especially for you and the particular problems you are experiencing.

Physical therapists rely on doctors, either your family physician or your neurologist, to send people with *PD* to them for treatment (this is called a referral).

Physical therapists can offer you better and longer lasting effects if they can be involved in your treatment before your movement becomes difficult.

If you or a family member have *PD,* ask your doctor or your neurologist for a referral to physiotherapy **right away!**

The physical therapist will keep your doctor fully informed of your progress in your program.

POSTURE

One of the major areas affected by *PD* is your **POSTURE** or the alignment of your body in standing or sitting (remember you teachers were always telling you to "Stand up straight!"). *PD* tends to make you bend over after some time, which can cause pain and interfere with your balance and walking. It can also cause difficulties in **BREATHING.** Your ribs are attached to your spine and help to make up a *cage* that surrounds your lungs. This cage moves as you breathe in and out and helps you to move more air through your lungs. A **"FLEXED POSTURE"** will interfere with the movement of this cage and this will eventually limit the movement of your lungs, which may cause you difficulty in breathing. Your lungs are very important parts of the body so we must prevent this from happening by maintaining the **CORRECT POSTURE** at all times.

EXERCISES: BREATHING

Improves movement of rib cage
You can do this exercise either standing, lying on the floor on your back, or sitting. Be sure to remember your **CORRECT POSTURE.**
Place you hands on your stomach, just below your ribs. Breathe from the bottom of your chest using a muscle called the diaphragm (helps you bring more air into your lungs).
When taking a breath in, your stomach will rise against your hands. Breathe in as far as you can, hold it for a second, and relax completely. The air will automatically leave your lungs. Repeat, slowly, three or four times, have a rest, and then do another set. Don't breathe too quickly or you will become dizzy.
You can also raise your arms above your head as you inhale, then lower them as you exhale.
Breathe **IN** through your nose and **OUT** through your mouth.
If you feel dizzy, stop and rest for a while. It probably means you are breathing too quickly.

EXERCISES: FACIAL MUSCLES

Improves muscles of facial expression and speech, which sometimes become stiff in *PD*. This can also affect your speech and eating.

REMEMBER **CORRECT POSTURE**
REMEMBER YOUR BREATHING
DO THESE EXERCISES IN FRONT OF A MIRROR

1. Wrinkle up forehead and nose and make a **big smile.** Show those teeth. Repeat ＿＿ times
2. Open mouth **wide** (making a big yawn or a silent roar). Repeat ＿＿ times
3. Squeeze your lips together (pucker for a kiss). Repeat ＿＿ times (whether someone takes you up on the offer or not!)

EXERCISES: ARMS

Improves range of movement of shoulders.

REMEMBER **CORRECT POSTURE**
REMEMBER YOUR BREATHING

1. Sitting or standing: grab a broom handle with both hands and raise arms up and over your head. Repeat ＿＿ times
2. Sitting or standing: bring arms up to shoulder height and make large circles. Repeat in both directions. Repeat ＿＿ times
3. Face a wall (about 8'' away); reach up wall as far as you can. Try to keep your palms on the wall. Repeat ＿＿ times

EXERCISES: LEGS

Improves range of movement at the hips and knees. ***PD*** can cause your hips and knees to bend.

REMEMBER **CORRECT POSTURE**
REMEMBER YOUR BREATHING

1. Sitting in a chair, put one leg on a small stool, stretch your trunk very gently and very slowly over that leg, and hold for a few seconds. Feel the nice **stretch.** Repeat with the other leg. Repeat ＿＿ times
2. Lie on you stomach without a pillow for about 15 minutes at a time. When this becomes easy, ease one leg up behind you for a moment, moving at your hip. Repeat with other leg. Repeat ＿＿ times
3. Hold onto the back of a chair and lift one leg out to the side. Repeat with the other leg. Repeat ＿＿ times

EXERCISES: TRUNK (BODY)

Improves movement of trunk, particularly your spine.

REMEMBER **CORRECT POSTURE**
REMEMBER YOUR BREATHING

1. Sitting on a stool, fold your arms across your chest and twist from side to side as far as you can without hurting yourself. Repeat ____ times
2. Standing with hands on your hips, twist at your waist to each side. Repeat ____ times
3. Standing: swing one arm out across your body while bringing the opposite leg forward. Repeat with each arm and leg. Repeat ____ times

BALANCE/WALKING

Your balance and walking pattern are very closely related, and often many exercises for one will benefit the other as well. ***PD*** can make you shuffle and take small steps.

Problems in these areas are common for people with ***PD.*** Causes for problems in these areas are due to both:

1. The disease itself
2. Medication

Balance has to be good so we can walk using as little energy as possible. Some problems are very common amongst people who have ***PD.*** Often you may find yourself:

1. Falling or tipping over
2. Shuffling and taking small steps
3. Having difficulty when trying to begin or stop walking

ALWAYS REMEMBER CORRECT POSTURE
REMEMEMBER YOUR BREATHING

TIPS FOR BETTER WALKING

Shuffling

1. Try to take longer steps
2. Lift your feet well off the ground with each step (exaggerate as if marching)
3. Try to always set your heel down on the ground first
4. Move your opposite arm with your opposite leg (i.e., right arm moves forward when left leg moves forward) (exaggerate arm swing)
5. If walking in home, it may help you to walk to music. Use a stereo, radio, or a Walkman (listen to music you enjoy).

If You Get Stuck, Try:

1. Rocking back and forth before taking a step
2. Make sure your heels are firmly on the ground and that you are not standing on your toes
3. Use a sound or look at something for a cue to start walking (e.g., say to yourself, **"On the count of three: one, two, THREE!"** trying a step on **THREE**), step over an imaginary line, or if an object is in front of you (crack on the side walk, a piece of garbage, or a small rock) then try to step over it.
4. Move a part of your body (e.g., swing your arms), then get your legs going (i.e., marching on the spot)
5. Try taking a step backward first

Improve Your Balance

1. Practice activities in which you can move or shift your weight around (e.g., dancing).
2. Walk with your legs slightly farther apart (about 10'' apart)
3. Make sure you keep the floor free from things you can trip over (throw rugs, kids' toys)

RELAXATION TECHNIQUES

Often people don't take "TIME OUT" from their daily lives to relax. Taking time to relax gives the body and the mind time to refresh themselves. **PD** can make the muscles tight and feel tired. Relaxing these muscles can often ease your discomfort. These techniques will help you to relax and they can be done whenever you feel you need to take "time out."

1. Find a comfortable position in which you can relax (if at home, you may lie down or, if at work, you may sit in a chair)
2. Try to find a quiet area where you aren't likely to be interrupted (you may even want to put on soft background music)
3. Turn out the lights
4. Close your eyes and try to erase your mind by concentrating on your breathing
5. Breathe slowly and regularly, saying to yourself, **"In and out"**
6. Beginning at your feet, tighten those muscles, hold them tight for a couple of seconds, and then let them go.
7. Next move to the muscles of your legs, tighten them, hold, and let go
8. Continue this all the way up to your facial muscles
9. When you have relaxed, think of pleasant memories or images that are relaxing.
10. You can do this as many times as you wish until you feel refreshed

HELPFUL HINTS

Try to lie on **your stomach** at least twice a day for about 10–15 minutes each time (this will help your posture)

Try to use your eyes when you are **walking.** Look for things on the ground or place objects on the ground so you will have to lift your feet to step over them

When rolling over in bed: bend up both knees, clasp your hands over your head and swing them from side to side until you have enough momentum to roll over. Be careful not to roll off the bed. You will need lots of room to roll

When getting up from a bed or chair, a high bed or chair with arm rests are the best.

Move to the **edge**

Place your feet **apart** and **behind** your knees

Begin rocking backwards and forwards

Aim to keep you **head up** and move it forward and upwards when you rise.

Look at something high up on a wall to keep your head right.

Count **"1, 2, 3, go!"**, and push up with arms and legs to standing.

If dressing becomes difficult try buying clothes with **zippers or velcro**

Break down your activities into steps, trying to **concentrate on one thing** at a time

Try to do activities in which you are **using your hands,** such as woodwork, knitting, crafts, etc.

WORK SHEET

Date of last assessment: ＿＿＿＿＿＿＿

Major areas to work on:

1.

2.

3.

4.

5.

Aims/Goals:

1.

2.

3.

4.

5.

Best time of day for exercising (at least 1/2 hr.): _____
List of activities to choose from at least 3 times per week:

1.

2.

3.

4.

5.

Remember, if you don't use it, you'll lose it.

8 | Physical Therapy Evaluation

Margaret H. Sharpe

Physiotherapy is frequently given to patients with Parkinson's disease (PD). However, objective methods for quantifying the patient's abilities and deficits, and the effects of therapeutic intervention, are seldom used.

Parkinson's disease has generally been considered a motor disorder. The classical triad of symptoms are bradykinesia,[1] rigidity,[1] and tremor.[2,3] Apart from these motor deficits, global intellectual deterioration has been reported in this clinical population,[4,5] as have more subtle and specific cognitive deficits affecting such capacities as memory,[6-8] language,[9] concept formation,[10-12] motor planning,[13-15] motor set,[16,17] visuospatial perception,[18] and attention.[19,20] As a consequence, it is imperative that the physical therapy evaluation take into account both the cognitive and motor deficits that have been widely reported in PD.

Since patients with PD have been shown to be distractible,[20] it is extremely important to conduct the evaluation in a quiet room without distractions.

Given the physiologic fluctuations related to PD and the medication used to treat it,[21] the physical therapist must always note the time of the last dose and the dosage of medication given, as well as the time of evaluation, so that all future evaluations are conducted at the same time of day.

The evaluation comprises two major parts: a subjective and an objective component. The information sought in the subjective evaluation is as follows:

Subjective evaluation
Psychosocial
Name
Age
Address
Date of admission (if hospitalized)

Date and time of evaluation
Marital status
Occupation (current and previous)
Interests/hobbies
Number of children
Degree of support from family and friends
Preferred hand
Mood
Patient's perceived needs, goals, issues
Patient's previous level of function, mobility, exercise tolerance, and fitness
Patient's premorbid intellectual and cognitive function
Medical history
Previous medical and surgical history
History of PD, treatment, and management
Ancillary investigations
Current medications
Orientation in time, place, and person
Current general health status

OBJECTIVE EVALUATION

Many clinical tests and scales may be used to identify and measure motor function in patients with PD. Some are quantitative and others qualitative.

Clinical Rating Scales

The advent of L-dopa therapy for PD has given rise to the development of clinical rating scales for the evaluation of motor impairment (tremor, rigidity, bradykinesia) and functional activities in the disease (see Marsden and Schachter[22] and Potvin and Tourtellote[23] for reviews). However, few attempts have been made to evaluate the reliability or validity of these scales, or to provide a rationale for the selection of their constituent items. The test items tend to fall into two categories: (1) sign and symptom items, which are formalizations of the tests used by neurologists to reveal parkinsonian impairment, and (2) activities of daily living items, which assess in a global fashion the functional status (including gait) of the patient. Nevertheless, Henderson and colleagues[24] have shown moderately high inter-rater reliability for these tests, with clinical experience having no systematic effect on ratings or their reliability. Moreover, their study also demonstrated that the major sources of unreliability appear to be inherent peculiarities and ambiguities in particular performances, rather than the expertise of the rater.

Tremor

Parkinsonian tremor may occur at rest or during action.[2,3] Several tests may be used to assess this motor deficit.

Static Steadiness Task for Resting Tremor

This test requires the patient to insert an electric stylus into circular holes of varying dimension. The patient is instructed to prevent the electric stylus from making contact with the sides of the hole. Errors are recorded by an electronic counter whenever the stylus makes contact with the sides of the hole.[25]

Maze Co-ordination Task for Action Tremor

This test requires the patient to complete a grooved maze with an electric stylus without touching the sides of the maze. Errors in which the sides are touched are recorded by an electronic counter.

Computerized Maze Co-ordination Task for Action Tremor

The patient is instructed to move a cursor, using a joystick or mouse, through a maze that is presented on a video monitor, and to avoid overshooting the boundaries. The total number of errors are scored, together with absolute errors and the time taken to correct an error. Timing, stimulus presentation, and data collection are under the programmed control of an IBM microcomputer.[25]

Bradykinesia

Bradykinesia describes a difficulty in initiating and sustaining voluntary movement. It may be observed in such functional activities of PD patients as handwriting, tying shoelaces, feeding, turning over in bed, walking, speech, and standing erect. The failure to produce fast ballistic movements is a striking and consistent feature of PD, even in its early stages.[26] The parkinsonian patient achieves movement by a repetitive series of small agonist-muscle activity bursts. This may be because the patient cannot achieve a sufficiently great initial burst in the agonist muscle despite the normal duration of the first agonist burst and preservation of the timing of subsequent antagonist and agonist bursts.[27] On the other hand, Sheridan and Flowers[28] have proposed that the difficulty of PD patients in moving lies not so much in the magnitude of the muscle force available to them, but rather in an inability to produce it consistently for any given movement.

Several different tasks may be employed to assess this motor deficit.

Finger- and Foot-Tapping Task

With this test, the patient is requested to tap a mechanical switch as quickly as possible using, either the index finger or foot.[29]

Computerized Tapping Task

Timing, stimulus presentation, and data collection for this task are under the programmed control of an IBM microcomputer.[30]

The patient is asked to repetitively tap a response switch as quickly as possible, using the index finger of each hand and foot in sequence, while seated. The number of responses, response latencies, and consistency of responses are recorded.

Grooved Pegboard

This task requires the patient to insert pegs into holes as quickly as possible. The patient's performance is timed.

Rigidity

Rigidity of muscles is a prominent feature of PD, and involves the axial and limb-girdle musculature before the distal segmental musculature. There is uniform resistance to passive movement throughout the whole range of motion at any joint, which is present to an equal degree in opposing muscle groups. This type of hypertonus is called *lead-pipe* rigidity. Another type of rigidity, *cogwheel* rigidity, is nonuniform resistance to passive movement throughout the whole range of motion at any joint, and has been attributed to a rhythmic interruption of the hypertonus by a coexisting resting or action tremor. Several clinical scales[31–34] based on ordinal measurement may be used to evaluate the absence or presence and the severity of rigidity in the musculature of the neck, trunk, and extremities.

Postural Control

The evaluation of standing balance is imperative for the treatment and management of instability in the PD patient. There is substantial evidence for abnormal postural control in these patients.[35–37]

Postural control relies on sensory information from the vestibular somato-sensory (proprioceptive, cutaneous, and joint), visual, and vestibular systems. Instability and other neurologic impairments in the PD patient[36-38] may result from inappropriate interaction among the three sensory inputs, which provide orientation information to the postural control system.[38-40] The PD patient has been shown to depend inappropriately on one sense for situations presenting intersensory conflict.[36]

It is therefore important for the therapist designing a therapeutic interven-tion program for the PD patient to determine the sense on which the patient is most dependent for sway orientation, and how well the patient may adapt (if at all) to reliance on each of the senses in situations of intersensory conflict.

This information may be obtained from the Sensory Organization Test (SOT) developed by Shumway-Cook and Horak.[41] The test requires the PD patient to maintain standing balance under six different intersensory conditions that either eliminate inputs or produce inaccurate visual and surface orientation inputs. Changes in the degree and direction of lateral and anteroposterior sway may be measured quantitatively using a shoulder harness developed by Shel-don.[42] The SOT has very high reliability.[43]

The Ataxia Test Battery

This test, developed by Graybiel and Fregly,[44] also quantitates postural control. There is a long and short version of the test. Both have normative values for men and women over a wide range of ages. Intratest and test-retest reliability have also been established and are moderately high. Details about the apparatus, administration, and scoring procedures for the long and short versions of the Ataxia Test battery are provided by Graybiel and Fregly.[44]

Movement Co-ordination Strategies

Apart from evaluating the sensory systems in PD patients, it is also im-portant to assess their movement co-ordination strategies. There are three strategies—ankle, hip, and stepping or stumbling[44a-c]—which have been shown to be impaired in this clinical population compared to normal adults.[44d]

Most frequently used is the ankle strategy. This enables the person to shift the body's center of gravity by rotating the body about the ankle joints with minimal hip and knee joint movement. In contrast, the hip strategy readjusts the center of gravity to hip flexion and extension. The stepping strategy realigns the base of support under the new position of the center of gravity with rapid hopping, stepping, or stumbling.[44a]

The configuration of the support surface and the magnitude of the perturba-tion determine the selection of a particular strategy. An ankle strategy is gener-ally used in response to slow, small perturbations on a firm, wide surface. Hip strategy is normally used in response to larger, faster perturbations on a compliant surface or a base smaller than the feet (i.e., standing crosswise on a narrow beam). This strategy must be avoided on slippery surfaces because hip sway transmits horizontal shear forces to the surface rather than vertical forces, as in the case of the ankle strategy. In response to very fast and large perturbations the stepping strategy is engaged because the hip and ankle strategies are inadequate. The selection of these movement co-ordination strategies seem to be based on previous experience. Evidence has shown that when the characteristics of the support surface are changed suddenly, normal adults initially use the same strategy but then switch to the new strategy, thus demonstrating a combination of two strategies before finally adopting the most efficient strategy for the new environmental context.[44a]

Motor Planning

Several studies have reported a motor planning deficit in PD patients.[13-15] To identify a motor planning deficit in the upper extremities, the Gestural Representation Test may be used.[45] This test is brief and easy to administer.

Gestural Test

There are two components to this test. The first component evaluates the level of gestural representation and involves the representation of implement usage (representational task). The second component is the imitation of nonrepresentational gestures (nonrepresentational task).

The representational task comprises 20 items, 10 of which are performed to verbal command and then repeated by imitation. For those items performed to verbal command, the patient is asked to represent the use of a specific implement (e.g., "Show me how you would eat with a spoon"). In contrast, for those items performed to imitation the patient is instructed to imitate the examiner, who demonstrates the use of each implement.

A further 10 items constitute the nonrepresentational task. On this task the subject is required to imitate hand and arm positions demonstrated by the examiner. The specific items for the representational and nonrepresentational tasks are shown in Tables 8-1 and 8-2, respectively.

Table 8-1. Representational Tasks on the Gestural Test

1. Show me how you would brush your teeth with a toothbrush
2. Show me how you would comb your hair with a comb
3. Show me how you would eat with a spoon
4. Show me how you would shave with a razor
5. Show me how you would smoke with a pipe
6. Show me how you would hit a nail with a hammer
7. Show me how you would turn a screw with a screwdriver
8. Show me how you would cut wood with a saw
9. Show me how you would cut paper with a scissors
10. Show me how you would make a hole in wood with a drill

Table 8-2. Nonrepresentational Tasks (to Imitation)

1. Dorsal side of hand covering ear, fingers extended and adducted (forearm supinated)
2. Thumb abducted to 90° and placed 0.5 in. from nose (fingers extended and adducted). Thumb maintains this position while hand is moved forward and backward over forehead three times in a rocking motion in the sagittal plane
3. Dorsal side of hand under chin, fingers extended and adducted
4. Hand to side of nose (fingers extended and adducted), palmar side medial
5. Arm out sideways, with arm externally rotated and abducted to 90°, forearm pronated and elbow flexed to 90°, wrist fully flexed and ulnar deviated
6. Arm out sideways, internally rotated and abducted to 90°, thumb abducted and pointing down with fingers extended and adducted, back of hand facing subject
7. Fingers 1 and 4 touching (palm down); other fingers extended and oriented to subject
8. Fingers 2 through 5 flexed to 90° at metacarpal joint and held extended and adducted. Thumb flexed at metacarpal joint and held extended 0.5 in. from finger 2. Hand positioned so that extended fingers are horizontal, parallel to and held about 1 ft. from mouth. Hand is moved from right to left and back three times with an 18-in. excursion
9. Beginning with hand held with palm toward self, arm makes three counterclockwise circles away from body, ending with arm extended and forearm supinated
10. Fingers 1 and 2 touching to form a circle (forearm neutral). Rest of fingers slightly flexed. Hand is moved outward toward subject to and from nose (without touching nose) three times.

Procedure

The examiner and patient sit facing each other with a table between them in a quiet room with no distractions. Representational and nonrepresentational items are presented only once. The representational items to be done to verbal command always precede the items to be done by imitation.

For the times on the representational items to verbal command, the examiner instructs the patient to pretend to be holding in the hand and using the tool that the examiner requests. To assure that the patient understands the instructions, a sample item is administered. On the representational and nonrepresentational items to imitation, the patient is required to imitate the hand and arm positions performed by the examiner.

Scoring

The representational items in the Gestural Test are scored for the developmental level of the gesture as well as for the number and type of spatial errors. The level of gesture for the representational items is determined by using Kaplan's[46] categories as follows:

1 point: Diectic Behavior (DB). The response focuses entirely on the action demonstrated, by either pointing to the implement or pointing to the object of action and thus locating where the action would occur (e.g., pointing to the mouth for "brushing teeth").

2 points: Body Part-object (BPO). The implement and characteristic action of the implement are represented by the body part. The patient positions part of his or her body in such a way as to ideally represent the perceptual, formal, physiognomic properties of the stimulus implement. The movement performed is the characteristic movement that the implement makes when it is manipulated by an agent (e.g., using the extended forefinger as the tooth-brush and making brushing movements against the teeth).

3 points: Holding Without Extent (H-E). The agent (body part) and the implement are differentiated, but the hand holding the implement is too close to the object of action (e.g., the hand holds the toothbrush but is held too close to the mouth).

4 points: Holding With Extent (H+E). The agent, implement, and object of action are fully differentiated. The patient holds the implement at a sufficient distance from the object of the action to indicate the formal extent of the implement (e.g., the hand is held far enough away from the mouth to indicate toothbrushing).

If the subject modifies his or her response, a half-point is either added or subtracted, depending on whether the change is to a higher or a lower level of gesture.

The nonrepresentational tasks are not scored for level of gesture. These items are scored only according to number and type of spatial errors. Spatial errors are also recorded for the representational items performed "to imitation." There are five possible types of spatial errors.

Location: Erroneous location either on the body or in extrapersonal space.
Plane: Any disorientation in plane for positioning of fingers, limbs, or body, or the orientation of movement through space.
Reversal: The reversal of movement in the anteroposterior plane.
Right-left: Right-left disorientation or mirror movements.
Finger position: Substitution of incorrect fingers when imitating the examiner's position.

Two scores are obtained: the total number of spatial errors on the 10 nonrepresentational items and the total number of spatial errors on the 10 representational items to imitation.

Axial Apraxia

Lakke[13] has proposed that the disorder of axial movement observed in PD is an apraxic phenomenon rather than an akinetic mechanism. The main evidence for this concept is derived from axial rotatory deficiencies (rolling over) and, to a lesser degree, from abnormalities seen in rising, kneeling, standing up, and walking. An evaluation of axial apraxia may be obtained from Lakke's[13] report.

Respiratory Function

Respiratory problems are a major cause of death in PD patients.[46] Most patients do not report respiratory problems, probably because their physical disability does not lead them to activities in which such problems may manifest themselves.

Several studies have reported respiratory abnormalities including upper airway obstruction,[47,48] coexisting chronic obstructive lung disease[49] due to increased bronchial muscle tone as a result of increased parasympathetic activity,[50] and decreased effective strength of the respiratory muscles in patients with parkinsonism and PD.[47]

It is possible to detect subclinical abnormalities and to localize them using modern methods of evaluating pulmonary function that are relatively easy to administer, noninvasive, and sensitive.

Pulmonary function testing would entail the evaluation of:

Vital capacity

Forced expiratory volume in 1 second

Maximum expiratory and maximal inspiratory flow-curves. The flow-volume curve (Fig 8-1) relates maximal expiratory and inspiratory flows to displaced volume during expiration and inspiration, respectively, and may be used to derive the following variables:

Peak expiratory flow

Peak inspiratory flow

Forced vital capacity

Forced inspiratory vital capacity

Forced inspiratory volume in 1 second

The ratios for forced expiratory volume 1sec/vital capacity, and maximal expiratory flow 50 percent/maximal inspiratory flow 50 percent.

Maximum expiratory flow 50 percent and maximum expiratory flow 25 percent may be calculated from the forced vital capacity, and represent the flow rate when 50 percent and 25 percent, respectively, of air remains in the lungs.

Maximum static mouth pressure at residual volume and total lung capacity may be measured according to the protocol of Black and Hyatt.[51]

Swallowing

Numerous studies have reported swallowing disorders in PD.[52-56] Lieberman and associates have found that dysphagia as assessed by barium swallow may be present in as many as 50 percent of patients with the disease.[54] Silbiger and co-workers have described the characteristic radiographic features of the parkinsonian swallow, including tongue tremor, hesitancy in initiating swallowing, difficulty in bolus formation, and disturbances in pharyngeal mobility.[56]

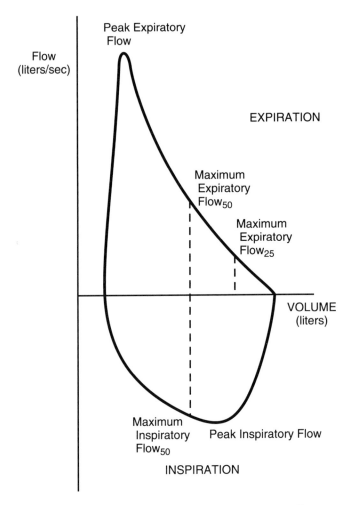

Fig. 8-1.   Flow-volume curve. (Adapted from Hovestadt et al.,[47] with permission.)

Furthermore, Robbins and associates,[57] using videofluoroscopy, have observed abnormal oropharyngeal movement patterns and timing during the oral as well as the pharyngeal stage of swallowing. They have suggested that rigidity and bradykinesia underlie disordered oral and pharyngeal swallowing. More importantly, their findings indicate that PD patients may be "silent aspirators" with decreased cough reflexes and lack of awareness of aspiration. This may explain the role of bronchopneumonia as a leading cause of death in PD.[46]

Because of such effects, it is important for the physical therapist to evaluate swallowing dysfunctions in PD patients, since the identification of aspiration at an early stage, when compensatory strategies may be attempted to prevent pneumonia, may be lifesaving.

A comprehensive evaluation of dysphagia for physical therapists has been designed by Cherney, Cantieri and Pannell.[58]

Gait

Although objective methods such as electrogoniometry, electromyography, force plates, and cinematography have been developed for obtaining quantitative information about gait, they are not easily used in the clinical setting because of equipment cost, space requirements, and the time needed to use them in testing. As a consequence, gait evaluation is based mainly on clinical observations, which may become an art with continued practice and application.

However, Robinson and Smidt[59] have developed a simple, economical technique that requires minimal equipment for quantifying the characteristics of the gait pattern. The four basic temporal and distance characteristics of gait that are quantifiable are velocity, cadence, stride length, and step length. They have been used in studies of normal and abnormal gait. Further information about the apparatus, procedure, and data analysis used in their gait measurement technique may be obtained from Robinson and Smidt.

Musculoskeletal System

Posture, range of joint motion, muscle strength, and extensibility need to be evaluated to prevent or minimize musculoskeletal limitations and postural deformities that may accompany PD, thereby limiting the patient's functional capacity, independence, and quality of life. Quantitative evaluation procedures for posture and the musculoskeletal system are clearly described by Kendall and McCreary[60] and Kendall.[61]

Motor Set

Patients with PD have difficulty in co-ordinating two or more movements.[16,17] In addition to exhibiting abnormalities in initiating individual movements and executing them (bradykinesia, hypokinesia), they appear to be unable to perform two tasks simultaneously,[62-64] to execute two or more sequential actions,[65-67] or to generate continuous movements without visual guidance.[68,69] These difficulties in co-ordination appear to involve the maintenance of a sequence of actions if two different actions are learned, requiring the patient to switch spontaneously from one to another.[16] Thus, PD patients show an impairment in motor set similar to that found previously in their cognitive activity. They perform better, however, if external cues are given to guide the ordering of movements at the start of each sequence.

Motor set may be easily evaluated by asking the PD patient to make a series of discrete movements in a given order in various repetitive sequences. By introducing a visual cue immediately before the motor sequences, the therapist will be able to determine whether the patient's ability to maintain or switch between motor sets improves.

Switching Attention

It has been suggested that PD patients have difficulty in switching cognitive set[13,70] and are more impaired when required to rely on internal attentional compared to external attentional control.[19]

This impaired ability to switch or shift attention has also been observed in bimanual simultaneous and repetitive motor tasks as compared to unimanual tasks. However the performance of PD patients on these bilateral tasks is improved with the use of external cues.[70] With this in mind, the therapist may instruct the PD patient to execute two functional motor tasks simultaneously with and without external (visual, auditory, tactile) cues to evaluate the patient's manual motor performance.

Unimanual functional motor tasks must be administered before the bimanual tasks to ensure that the patient has no difficulty with separate unimanual tasks.

Predictive Control of Movement

Evidence suggests that PD patients fail to engage the normal strategies of prediction during visual tasks, and are therefore unable to utilize an "internal model" of external events when executing motor activities. This results in a loss of visual-motor skills, which leads to a greater dependency on sensory and especially visual information.[68] The failure to employ a predictive strategy imposes considerable constraints on motor performance, to the extent that the patient relies on external cues and feedback from the execution of movements, which in turn prevents the execution of movements more rapid than the limits imposed by reaction time (RT).

Predictive or anticipatory voluntary movement may be evaluated by placing the patient in an open environment (e.g., walking in an unfamiliar and crowded street, catching a ball, hitting a balloon, negotiating an obstacle course).[71]

Computerized Visual Tracking Task

This task requires the PD patient to track a visual target through a known and an unknown path. The number of tracking errors are recorded for both types of paths.

Timing, stimulus presentation, data collection and analysis are under the programmed control of an IBM microcomputer.[72]

REFERENCES

1. Lee RG: Pathophysiology of rigidity and akinesia in Parkinson's disease. Eur Neurol (suppl 1):513, 1989
2. Koller WC, Huber SJ: Tremor disorders of aging: diagnosis and management. Geriatrics 44:33, 1989

3. Koller WC, Vetere-Overfield B, Barter R: Tremors in early Parkinson's disease. Clin Neuropharmacol 12:293, 1989
4. Pirozzolo FJ, Hansch EC, Mortimer JA et al: Dementia in Parkinson's disease; neuropsychological analysis. Brain Cogn 1:71, 1982
5. Reitan RM, Boll RJ: Intellectual and cognitive function in Parkinson's disease. J Consult Clin Psychol 37:364, 1971
6. Tweedy JR, Langer KG, McDowell FH: The effect of semantic relations on the memory deficit associated with Parkinson's disease. J Clin Neuropsychol A:235, 1982
7. Flowers KA, Pearce I, Pearce JMS: Recognition memory in Parkinson's disease. J Neurol Neurosurg Psychiatry 47:1174, 1984
8. Morris RG, Downes JJ, Sahakian BJ et al: Planning and spatial working memory in Parkinson's disease. J Neurol Neurosurg Psychiatry 51:757, 1988
9. Matison R, Mayeux R, Rosen J, Fahn S: "Tip of the tongue" phenomenon in Parkinson disease. Neurology 32:567, 1982
10. Bowen FP, Kamienny RS, Burns MM, Yahr MD: Parkinsonism: effects of levedopa treatment on concept formation. Neurology 25:701, 1975
11. Flowers KA, Robertson C: The effect of Parkinson's disease on the ability to maintain a mental set. J Neurol Neurosurg Psychiatry 48:517, 1985
12. Lees AJ, Smith E: Cognitive deficits in the early stages of Parkinson's disease. Brain 106:257, 1983
13. Lakke JPWF: Axial apraxia in Parkinson's disease. J Neurol Sci 69:37, 1985
14. Goldenberg G, Wimmer A, Auff E, Schnaberth G: Impairment of motor planning in patients with Parkinson's disease: evidence from ideomotor apraxia testing. J Neurol Neurosurg Psychiatry 49:1266, 1986
15. Sharpe MH, Cermak SA, Sax DS: Motor planning in Parkinson patients. Neuropsychologia 21:455, 1983
16. Robertson C, Flowers KA: Motor set in Parkinson's disease. J Neurol Neurosurg Psychiatry 53:583, 1990
17. Brown RG, Marsden CD: An investigation of the phenomenon of "set" in Parkinson's disease. Mov Disord 3:152, 1988
18. Boller F, Passafiume D, Keefe NC et al: Visuospatial impairment in Parkinson's disease: role of perceptual and motor factors. Arch Neurol 41:485, 1984
19. Brown RG, Marsden CD: Internal versus external cues and the control of attention in Parkinson's disease. Brain 111:323, 1988
20. Sharpe MH: Distractibility in early Parkinson's disease. Cortex 26:239, 1990
21. Brown RG, Marsden CD, Quinn N, Wyke M: Alterations in cognitive performance and affect-arousal state fluctuations in motor function in Parkinson's disease. J Neurol Neurosurg Psychiatry 47:454, 1984
22. Marsden CD, Schachter M: Assessment of extrapyramidal disorders. Br J Clin Pharmacol 11:129, 1981
23. Potvin PE, Tourtellotte MD: Quantitative Examination of Neurological Function. CRC Press, Boca Raton, Florida, 1984
24. Henderson L, Kennard C, Crawford TJ et al: Scales for rating motor impairment in Parkinson's disease: studies of reliability and covergent validity. J Neurol Neurosurg Psychiatry 54:18, 1991
25. Sharpe MH, Williams D: Computerised maze co-ordination task. University of South Australia, 1991
26. Wilson SAK: Disorders of mobility and muscle tone, with special reference to the striatum. Lancet 2:1, 169, 215, 268, 1925

27. Hallet M, Koshbin S: A physiological mechanism of bradykinesia. Brain 103:301, 1980
28. Sheridan MR, Flowers KA: Movement variability and bradykinesia in Parkinson's disease. Brain 113:1149, 1990
29. Van Buren JM, Choh-Luh L, Shapiro Y et al: A qualitative and quantitative evaluation of Parkinsonians three to six years following thalotomy. Conf Neurol 35:202, 197327
30. Sharpe MH, Williams D: Computerised tapping task. University of South Australia, 1991
31. Webster DD: Critical analysis of the disability in parkinson's disease. Mod Treat 5:257, 1968
32. Lieberman AN: Parkinson's disease: a clinical review. Am J Med Sci 267:66, 1974
33. Lesser RP, Fahn S, Snider S et al: Analysis of clinical problems in parkinsonism and the complication of long-term levodopa therapy. Neurology 29:253, 1979
34. Canter GL, de la Torre R, Mier M: A method for evaluating disability in patients with Parkinson's disease. J Nerv Ment Dis 133:143, 1961
35. Purdon-Martin J: The Basal Ganglia and Posture. JB Lippincott, Philadelphia, 1967
36. Bronstein AM, Hood JD, Gresty MA et al: Visual control of balance in cerebellar and parkinsonian syndromes. Brain 113:767, 1990
37. Reichert WH, Doolittle, J, McDowell FH: Vestibular dysfunction in Parkinson's disease. Neurology 32:1133, 1982
38. Nashner CM, Black FO, Wall C: Adaptation to altered support and visual conditions during stance. Patients with vestibular deficits. J Neurosci 2:536, 1982
39. Nashner LM, Shumway-Cook A, Marin O: Stance posture control in select groups of children with cerebral palsy: deficits in sensory organization and muscular coordination. Exp Brain Res 49:393, 1983
40. Nashner LM, Black FO: Effect of abnormal vestibular-visual interaction upon posture control in two different types of vestibular deficit patients. Soc Neurosci Abstr 9:317, 1983
41. Shumway-Cook A, Horak FB: Assessing the influence of sensory interaction on balance. Phys Ther 66:1548, 1983
42. Sheldon JH: The effect of age on the control of sway. Gerontologica 5:129, 1963
43. Bamford E, Sharpe MH: Test-retest reliability of the sensory organization test (manuscript in preparation).
44. Graybiel A, Fregly AR: A new quantitative ataxia test battery. Acta Otolaryngol 61:293, 1966
44a. Horak FB, Nashner LM: Central programming of postural movements: adaptation to altered support surface configurations. J Neurophysiol 55:1369, 1986
44b. Nashner LM, McCollum G: The organization of human postural movements: a formal basis and experimental synthesis. Behav Brain Sci 8:135, 1985
44c. Wolfson LI, Whipple R, Amerman P, Kleinberg A: Stressing the postural response: a quantitative method for testing balance. J Am Geriatr Soc 34:845, 1986
44d. Horak FB, Nashner LM, Nutt J: Postural instability in parkinsonian patients: role of basal ganglia in postural strategies. Soc Neurosci Abstr 10:604, 1984
45. Kaplan E: Gestural representation of implement usage: an organismic-developmental study. Unpublished doctoral dissertation, Clark University, Worcester, Massachusetts, 1968
46. Hoehn MM, Yahr MD: Parkinsonism: onset, progression and mortality. Neurology 17:427, 1967
47. Hovestadt A, Bogaard JM, Meerwaldt JD, Van der Meché FGA: Pulmonary function in Parkinson's disease. J Neurol Neurosurg Psychiatry 52:329, 1989

48. Vincken W, Gauthier SG, Dolfuss RE et al: Involvement of upper airway muscles in extrapyramidal disorders; a cause of airflow irritation. N Engl J Med 311:438, 1984
49. Neu HC, Connolly JJ, Schwertly FW et al: Obstructive respiratory dysfunction in parkinsonian patients. Am Rev Resp Dis 95:33, 1967
50. Obenour WH, Stevens PM, Cohen AA, McCutchen JJ: The causes of abnormal pulmonary function in Parkinson's disease. Am Rev Resp Dis 105:382, 1972
51. Black LF, Hyatt RE: Maximal respiratory pressures: normal values and relationship to age and sex. Am Rev Resp Dis 99:699, 1969
52. Blonsky ER, Logemann JA, Boshes B, Fisher HB: Comparison of speech and swallowing function in patients with tremor disorders and in normal geriatric patients: a cinefluorographic study. J Gerontol 30:299, 1975
53. Calne DM, Shaw DG, Spiers AS, Stern GM: Swallowing in parkinsonism. Br J Radiol 43:456, 1970
54. Lieberman AN, Hirowitz L, Redmond P: Dysphagia in Parkinson's disease. Am J Gastroenterol 74:157, 1980
55. Palmer ED: Dsyphagia in parkinsonism. JAMA 229:1349, 1974
56. Silbiger MC, Pikielney R, Donner MW: Neuromuscular disorders affecting the pharynx: cineradiographic analysis. Invest Radiol 2:442, 1967
57. Robbins JA, Logemann JA, Kirshner H: Swallowing and speech production in Parkinson's disease. Ann Neurol 19:283, 1986
58. Cherney LR, Cantieri CA, Pannell JJ: Clinical Evaluation of Dysphagia. Rehabilitation Institute of Chicago. CED Aspen Publishers, Inc, Chicago, 1986
59. Robinson JL, Smidt GL: Quantitative gait evaluation in the clinic. Phys Ther 61:351, 1981
60. Kendall FP, McCreary EK: Muscles, Testing and Function. 3rd Ed. Williams & Wilkins, Baltimore, 1983
61. Kendall HO: Posture and Pain. Williams & Wilkins, Baltimore, 1983
62. Schwab RS, Chafetz ME, Walker S: Control of two simultaneous voluntary acts in normals and in parkinsonism. Arch Neurol Psychiatry 72:591, 1954
63. Talland GA, Schwab RS: Performance with multiple sets in Parkinson's disease. Neuropsychologia 2:45, 1964
64. Benecke R, Rothwell JC, Dick JPR et al: Performance of simultaneous movements in patients with Parkinson's disease. Brain 109:739, 1986
65. Schwab RS, Zieper I: Effects of mood, motivation, stress and alertness on the performance in Parkinson's disease. Psychiatr Neurol (Basel) 150:345, 1965
66. Flowers KA: Some frequency response characteristics of parkinsonism on pursuit tracking. Brain 101:19, 1978
67. Benecke R, Rothwell JC, Dick JPR et al: Disturbance of sequential movements in patients with Parkinson's disease. Brain 110:361, 1987
68. Flowers KA: Lack of prediction in the motor behaviour of Parkinsonism. Brain 101:35, 1978
69. Stern Y, Mayeux R, Rosen J, Ilson J: Perceptual motor dysfunction in Parkinson's disease: a deficit in sequential and predictive voluntary movement. J Neurol Neurosurg Psychiatry 46:145, 1983
70. Horstink MWIM, Berger HJC, van Spaendock KPM et al: Bimanual simultaneous motor performance and impaired ability to shift attention in Parkinson's disease. J Neurol Neurosurg Psychiatry 53:685, 1990
71. Poulton EC: On prediction in skilled movements. Psychol Bull 54:467, 1957
72. Sharpe MH, Williams D: Computerised visual tracking task. University of South Australia, 1991

9 | Physical Therapy Intervention for the Ambulatory Patient

Margaret Schenkman

This chapter provides an approach to physical therapy management of patients early in the course of Parkinson's disease (PD). Its focus is on management of the ambulatory patient from the time of initial diagnosis of PD throughout the period that the patient remains independently mobile. Much of the material in this chapter can also be applied to patients in later stages of the disease, after significant dependence occurs, although the particular problems of the functionally dependent patient are not addressed here.

The diagnosis of PD is generally made some time after the initial symptoms have appeared. By the time a definitive diagnosis of the disease can be made, the patient generally has some evidence of tremor, rigidity, and slowness of movement.[1-3] Postural alterations, altered gait patterns, and loss of facial expression may also be apparent. The afflicted individual may have observed these changes over a period of years before the diagnosis of PD.

Once the initial medical diagnosis of PD is made, the progression and manifestations of the disease vary considerably. Some patients have significant postural alterations and rigidity early in the disease; for others, tremor predominates. For some, the course of the disease is slow, with disability developing gradually, over a period of years or decades. For others, the period between initial diagnosis and total dependence can be shorter.[2]

The PD patient eventually and inevitably becomes significantly disabled.[1-3] Typical physical disabilities are evident in all phases of daily activity. Gross motor skills such as bed mobility, coming to a standing from a sitting position, and gait can become difficult or impossible. Fine motor skills such as writing, eating, and speaking are likewise affected. Respiratory dysfunction occurs, with pneumonia being a leading cause of death for the PD patient.[2,4]

These physical disabilities may lead to social withdrawal and isolation, and may contribute to depression, which frequently accompanies PD. Mental disturbances are also associated with PD, although there is a continuing debate in the literature about whether these mental alterations are a direct effect of the disease process itself, are changes associated with the normal aging process, or are a side effect of the pharmacologic agents used to treat the disease.[5,6]

Physical therapy intervention for the PD patient can neither stop nor retard the neuropathologic changes that occur in the disease. Such intervention can, however, improve the quality of life of the PD patient within the context of the disease. The purpose of physical therapy intervention early in the disease process is to reduce or retard the onset of physical disabilities through management of the underlying impairments. Early physical therapy intervention, in conjunction with medical management, can potentially delay the onset of physical disabilities, may delay the need for pharmacologic intervention, and perhaps most important can provide the patient with some control over his or her life despite the disease.[7]

This chapter provides the reader with both a philosophy and specific guidelines for management of the PD patient early in the disease process. Typical problems of PD are presented. A systematic approach for analyzing and interpreting the causes of these problems is then described. Appropriate goals are discussed, based on that analysis. Specific suggestions are then presented for patient evaluation and treatment.

PROBLEMS AND APPROACH TO PHYSICAL THERAPY INTERVENTION

An Overview of Problems

Tremor and rigidity (or stiffness) are the most frequent early signs of PD.[2] Both may interfere with dexterity and fine motor skills, such as writing and manual capability.[1] Rigidity is generally apparent in the upper body before it is evident in the lower extremities. Loss of facial expression is another early sign of PD, frequently causing the affected individual to appear distressed, worried, or anxious, and sometimes resulting in a misdiagnosis of psychiatric disorder. Changes in the voice may also be evident early in the disease. Initially there may be an apparent hoarseness, and later the voice may become progressively softer until it is hard to hear.[1]

Musculoskeletal alterations also begin to appear early in PD, eventually resulting in the stooped, flexed posture with extreme forward head carriage that characterizes PD. These postural and musculoskeletal alterations may first appear unilaterally, resulting on a scoliosis.[1] Scoliosis seems to occur early in the disease, when rigidity is more severe unilaterally. The postural alterations, coupled with immobility and accelerated degenerative changes, may result in pain, particularly of the shoulder.

As the disease progresses, other symptoms begin to appear,[1,2] including a delay in the initiation of movement, a general slowing of all movements, and a breakdown in the capability for motor planning. Functional movements such as mobility in bed, rising to standing from a seated position, and gait all become increasingly affected. The spontaneous movements normally associated with functional activities begin to disappear. For example, reciprocal arm swinging no longer occurs during gait, and the face is expressionless during speaking. Balance is gradually affected, contributing to the difficulty in performing all functional tasks. Furthermore, dystonic movements may occur as a side effect of pharmacologic agents used to treat the disease. These dystonic movements can interfere with all aspects of function.

A number of investigators have developed scales to characterize the progression and degree of disability from PD.[2,8-10] The Hoehn and Yahr stage of disease, New York University disability scale, and Northwestern University disability scale are among those that are most frequently cited in the literature.[10] These scales differ with respect to the emphasis that each places on various aspects of the disease.[10] The scale of Hoehn and Yahr, for example, emphasizes the interrelationship of balance disturbance and disability. The New York University disability scale rates rigidity, tremor, bradykinesia, gait, and postural stability. The Northwestern University disability scale emphasizes activities of daily living.[10]

Because the scoring systems used to grade PD differ in focus, the clinician may have difficulty definitively characterizing a patient's disease stage. Furthermore, there is great variability in the presentation of symptoms of PD, contributing to the difficulty in classifying the severity of disease for a particular patient. For purposes of this chapter, early stages of PD refer to Stages 1–3 of Hoehn and Yahr.[2] These authors broadly characterize patients as being in Stage 1 if they have unilateral involvement with minimal or no functional involvement; in Stage 2 if they have bilateral or midline involvement without balance impairment; in Stage 3 if they have impaired righting reflexes (balance) with some restriction in functional activity but with the capacity for living independent lives; in Stage 4 if they have severely incapacitating disease but are still able to walk and stand without assistance; and in Stage 5 if they are confined to a bed and a wheelchair except when assisted.

The diagnosis of PD generally is not made while patients are in Stage 1. Those in Stages 2 and 3 (when diagnosis of the disease is made) have increasing numbers of problems associated with the disease, but remain able to carry out relatively normal lives. By Stage 4, patients are beginning to experience disability in some or all aspects of their life, and in Stage 5, they are severely and totally disabled. As the disease progresses, social, emotional, and mental disabilities occur in addition to physical disability. As patients become physically disabled, there is a tendency for social withdrawal. For example, they report that their tendency to drool while eating, their difficulty with voice production, and their lack of facial expression can all lead to social isolation.

Lack of movement limits the PD patient's engagement in normal social interactions, further contributing to isolation. Social isolation can easily lead to depression.

The PD patient's problems that are treated by physical therapists can be characterized as stemming from three broad categories: motor-control abnormalities, musculoskeletal abnormalities, and cardiopulmonary abnormalities. Motor-control abnormalities include rigidity, tremor, and deficits in motor planning. Musculoskeletal abnormalities include loss of vertebral and limb segmental mobility as well as malalignment. Cardiopulmonary abnormalities include decreased cardiovascular endurance and decreased pulmonary function. Evidence of problems in each of these areas can be apparent in the early stages of PD.

The physical therapy intervention discussed in this chapter is directed toward persons in Stages 2 and 3 of Hoehn and Yahr. The goals of physical therapy intervention, while PD patients are still functionally able and independent, are as follows:

1. To teach patients strategies for self-management of those impairments of neurologic origin that are directly caused by the disease (e.g., rigidity, tremor, motor-planning difficulties), in order to reduce the impact of these impairments on their lives.

2. To prevent or retard the onset of impairments caused indirectly by the disease (e.g., musculoskeletal, respiratory, and cardiopulmonary problems).

3. To provide patients and their families with physical techniques that will assist the patient to delay the onset of physical, social, and emotional disabilities associated with the disease.

Philosophical Approach Toward Intervention

The general approach toward intervention presented in this chapter is based on a combination of motor control issues with mechanical and kinesiologic realities. These two aspects of the treatment approach to PD are outlined here to establish the focus of the remainder of this chapter.

The term motor control is used in this chapter to refer to impairments of motor planning, timing, initiation of movement, rigidity, tremor, and postural stability mechanisms. Deficits in these areas can be a direct result of the neurologic degeneration in PD.[11,12] Once the causes and consequences of these impairments are identified for a particular patient, the clinician can make decisions about whether these impairments can themselves be corrected or whether the emphasis of treatment should be on preventing the sequelae that result from these deficits. The thought process used to make this decision during the care of particular patients is outlined in the section of this chapter on the cause and effect of PD.

In this chapter, motor behaviors are identified as voluntary or reflexive, as

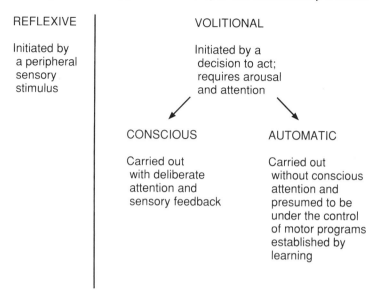

REFLEXIVE | VOLITIONAL

Initiated by
a peripheral
sensory
stimulus

Initiated by a
decision to act;
requires arousal
and attention

CONSCIOUS   AUTOMATIC

Carried out
with deliberate
attention and
sensory feedback

Carried out
without conscious
attention and
presumed to be
under the control
of motor programs
established by
learning

Fig. 9-1. Three categories of motor behavior.

described previously by Schenkman and Butler[11,12] (Fig. 9-1). The term *voluntary motor behaviors* refers to postures and movements that are initiated by the person's own decision to act.[12-14] Voluntary motor behaviors are differentiated into *conscious* and *automatic* components. Conscious motor behaviors are those components of voluntary motor behaviors that are carried out under deliberate control, with attention and deliberate correction. Many of the exercises done by the PD patient are performed with attention to the evolving movement patterns and correction as appropriate. Exercises done in this way fall into the category of conscious motor behavior. One example is the familiar exercise of having a patient step in footprints that were previously placed on the floor.[15] The components of the motor behavior that include stepping into the footprints and correcting the foot placement are considered conscious motor behaviors for the purposes of this chapter.

A motor action can be called *automatic* when it is initiated deliberately (voluntarily) but is carried out without conscious attention to sensory feedback.[12-14] Most postural adjustments and balance responses that accompany voluntary movements fall into the category of automatic motor behaviors. These responses represent the component of a motor behavior that the person expressing the behavior does not think about and does not consciously execute or correct. When a patient locates his or her feet over footprints placed on the floor, there are many postural adjustments of the pelvis, trunk, neck, and upper extremites that occur automatically in synchrony with the conscious aspects of the motor task described above.

Finally, motor behaviors that are obligatory responses to peripheral sensory stimuli are called *reflexive*. Their initiation differs from that of voluntary motor behaviors in that they are not undertaken consciously through a decision to act, but instead occur in response to peripheral stimuli. Reflexive corrections of posture can accompany automatic adjustments during functional movements. These aspects of motor behavior are depicted in Figure 9-1. In this chapter, motor-control issues are differentiated into those that relate to conscious, automatic, and reflexive motor behaviors.

The term *mechanical and kinesiologic realities* is used in this chapter to refer to those limitations resulting from the PD patient's musculoskeletal alignment and mobility. The mechanical and kinesiologic aspects of intervention can best be demonstrated by a few examples. All human postures and movements are constrained by the laws of mechanics and by kinesiologic imperatives.[16] The laws of mechanics ultimately determine, for example, whether a person is stable and can remain upright, or is unstable and will fall. In ideal postures the body is aligned in such a way that the vertical projection of the force of gravity acting on the body (center of gravity [COG]) will fall within the support base and will pass close to the joint axes of motion.[17] In these postures, the moment arms produced by gravity acting at joint axes are minimized, and the forces of muscles required to keep the body upright are likewise minimized. In the extreme forward head posture, the center of mass (COM) of the head is positioned anterior to the hip, knee, and ankle joint axes of motion. The laws of mechanics dictate that if the COG moves far enough anteriorly to fall outside the base of support, an individual will fall unless other forces, such as inertial forces, are present.[16] Thus, when the head posture is excessively forward, there is a mechanical need to restore the COG within the base of support by some compensatory postural strategy. For example, the hips can be flexed and the buttocks shifted posteriorly (Fig. 9-2). In other words, typical parkinsonian postures can be analyzed to identify the mechanical relationships between observed alterations of postures from the ideal.

From a kinesiologic perspective, once mechanical alterations have been imposed on the body's structure, the action of muscles needed to accomplish a task must also be altered. Rolling over in bed can be used to illustrate this point. One strategy for accomplishing this maneuver is to use segmental rotation. The term segmental rotation is used to indicate that rotation occurs at many vertebral segments. The PD patient typically loses mobility throughout the cervical, thoracic, and lumbar spine. The patient may therefore be unable to roll over in bed by using segmental strategies of movement. Consequently, a PD patient may get out of bed by sitting straight up and pivoting on the buttocks to swing the legs over the side of the bed. Such a strategy puts great demands on the rectus abdominus muscle, while minimizing the more normal use of the abdominal oblique and erector spinae muscles that are used for trunk rotation.[18] In other words, the combination muscles that would normally work together to accomplish a task may be altered because the strategy used to accomplish the task is changed by mechanical limitations.

The PD patient's posture and movement should be analyzed from a mechanical and kinesiologic perspective to identify clearly the constraints on movement and to interpret the mechanical reasons for observed movement patterns. The

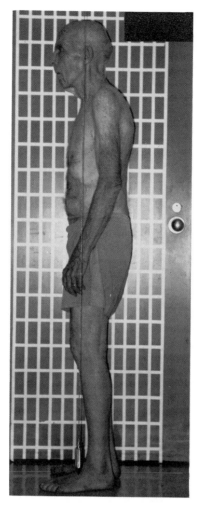

Fig. 9-2. Parkinsonian individual with forward head, flexed hips, and flexed knees, illustrating the combined postural deviations that may be necessary to preserve stability (From Schenkman,[16] with permission.)

heart of the interventional approach outlined in this chapter lies in coupling the mechanical observations of the patient with the motor-control issues affecting the patient to understand why the mechanical alterations have occurred and to decide how best to remediate them.

Treatment strategies can be developed from a synthesis of motor-control and mechanical issues. A mechanical and kinesiologic perspective of treatment can be illustrated by an example. One of the popular approaches to treatment of the neurologically impaired adult is the neurodevelopmental treatment (NDT) approach. This approach was originally founded on the premise that adult recovery from neurologic insults recapitulates infant development.[19] The assumptions underlying this approach have been brought into question[20] as more information has become available about the neurophysiology of the nervous system under normal and abnormal conditions. The approach itself can, however, be rationalized from a mechanical and kinesiologic perspective. The entire "developmental sequence" of activities begins with patients in the most supported positions that are mechanically least demanding, and progresses toward the least supported and mechanically more demanding postures. [In the supine position, the basis of support is large, and the center of mass (COM) of the body is low; in the standing position the base of support is small and the COM is high.) Furthermore, the developmental sequence progresses from kinesiologically simple to kinesiologically complex movements. Trunk rotation in sidelying is a kinesiologically simple movement in that it can be accomplished by the use of relatively few muscles working in synchrony (e.g., the thorax can be rotated on the pelvic complex by use of the abdominus oblique, the pectoralis, and cervical rotator muscles). There is limited requirement for muscles to stabilize the body against the force of gravity, because the body mass is supported on the bed of a treatment mat. In sitting, this same motion requires the coordinated participation of additional muscles (e.g., the erector spinae muscles and diverse muscles of the pelvic complex and neck) to stabilize the body against gravity and as helping and neutralizing synergists in the activity of trunk rotation. (Schenkman and Rugo de Cartaya[21] have provided a kinesiologic analysis of shoulder-complex motion that differentiates between muscles acting as movers, synergists, and stabilizers. This same kinesiologic approach can be applied to analyze any functional activity in order to identify all relevant components of a movement.)

Restoration of spinal mobility and function may be most efficiently accomplished if these mechanical and kinesiologic aspects of movement are interwoven into the treatment approach. It may be important to initiate treatment of a PD patient in fully supported positions even when the patient is completely independent in his or her daily life. These fully supported positions permit both the therapist and the patient to focus on restoration of mobility at every spinal segment and in every plane of movement. They also allow the therapist and patient to restore coordinated muscle action by working progressively from the simplest combinations of muscles to increasingly complex combinations.

The treatment approach outlined in this chapter interrelates treatment from a mechanical and kinesiologic perspective with treatment from a motor-control perspective. Neither approach can stand on its own in management of the PD patient; both are essential.

THE RELATIONSHIP BETWEEN CAUSE AND EFFECT IN PARKINSON'S DISEASE

Why Analyze Cause and Effect?

Physical therapy in PD will be most effective if intervention is based on a clear understanding of the neurologic disease process itself, the sequelae that result both directly and indirectly from the neurologic insult, and the interrelationship between the patient's problems and his or her own lifestyle and goals. An understanding of the relationship between cause and effect can aid the clinician in two ways: first, by permitting treatment to be directed at causes rather than symptoms; second, by permitting the clinician to make educated decisions about which problems to attempt to correct, which to compensate for, and which to prevent. These decisions are particularly necessary when treating patients with chronic degenerative diseases in which total disability is a probable eventual outcome.

In PD, the patient's eventual disability generally occurs because of the combined effect of many problems associated with the disease. A model developed by Schenkman and Butler[11,12] can be used for analyzing the contributions of various problems (e.g., rigidity, tremor, bradykinesia, postural abnormalities, and loss of range of motion) to the patient's loss of function. The model allows the clinician to interpret the PD patient's problems from the current theories of motor control, neurophysiology, kinesiology, and biomechanics. The model provides a system for integrating neurologic and non-neurologic problems in interpreting the patient's functional losses.

Elements of the Model on which Intervention is Based

In Schenkman and Butler's model,[11,12] a distinction is made between disability, impairments, and pathology. *Disability* refers to the inability to function within the range of normal. Disabilities may be physical, social, emotional, or mental.[22,23] The PD patient may experience disabilities in each of these areas. Loss of capability for independent or normal function in any area of daily life represents a physical disability. The ultimate goal of physical therapeutic intervention is to restore or maintain physical activity. The isolation and withdrawal associated with PD represent social disabilities. Depression can become an emotional disability, and dementia represents a mental disability. Clinicians who treat PD patients are faced with the task of interpreting the particular causes that are most responsible for the patients' observed disabilities. Thus, the clinician who treats a physical disability such as a gait disorder attempts to elucidate the underlying causes of that disorder. The term *impairment* refers to abnormalities of function of specific systems of the body, such as the neurologic, musculoskeletal, and cardiopulmonary systems. Impairments are the underlying causes of disabilities. Disorders of gait can be used to illustrate this concept. Impairments such as rigidity, bradykinesia, loss of mobility, and postural deviations can all potentially contribute to a gait disability. Often the clinician focuses intervention at specific impairments as a means of effectively treating disabilities.

Impairments associated with neurologic disorders are caused by *pathology*. The neuroanatomic pathology of PD affects neurotransmitters in the brainstem, basal ganglia, and cortex,[24,25] and is increasingly well understood. A knowledge of the neuroanatomic pathology of PD can be used to predict which impairments will result and to interpret the expected disabilities.

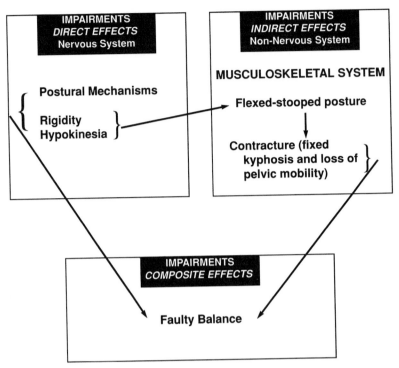

Fig. 9-3. Poor balance may be a composite effect of the neuroanatomic pathology of PD. (Reprinted from Schenkman and Butler[12] with permission.)

Impairments may result directly or indirectly from PD.[12] An analysis of gait can be used to illustrate this concept. Some impairments that underlie abnormal gait, such as rigidity and poor motor planning, are *direct effects* of the neuroanatomic pathology of the disease. That is, these impairments are the direct and specific result of the neuroanatomic destruction inherent in the disease. Impairments that are direct effects of PD, such as rigidity and tremor, may be ameliorated by pharmacologic intervention.[26] These impairments are unlikely to be prevented by physical therapy management, because they are a direct result of neurologic destruction. Other impairments, such as loss of range of motion, are an *indirect effect* of the neuroanatomic pathology of PD. That is, loss of intervertebral segmental mobility and malalignment in PD are not caused directly by the neuroanatomic pathology of the disease. Rather, these impairments are sequelae that could result from its direct effects (e.g., ensuing rigidity and lack of initiation of movement).[11,27] Because these indirect effects of the disease are not specifically linked to its neuroanatomic pathology, it may be possible to prevent or correct them through appropriate physical therapy management.

Certain impairments that affect gait may be *composite effects* of the neuroanatomic pathology in PD. Poor balance and bradykinesia, for example, might both contribute to a gait disability. Furthermore, both of these impairments might themselves be composite effects of PD (Fig. 9-3 and 9-4) Poor balance

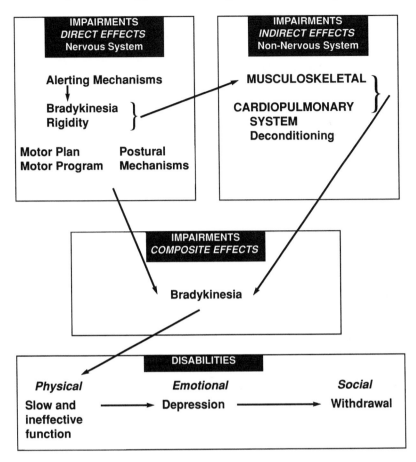

Fig. 9-4.   Bradykinesia may be a composite effect of PD. (From Schenkman and Butler,[12] with permission.)

may result from a combination of rigidity, poor motor planning, and loss of joint range of motion and malalignment. Rigidity and poor motor planning can be considered direct effects of PD, while loss of joint range of motion and malalignment can be considered indirect effects of the disease. Losses of postural response mechanisms that are a direct effect of the neuroanatomic destruction in PD may not be corrected through physical therapy management. Impairment of balance control due to malalignment and loss of joint mobility may, however, be corrected through physical techniques. Thus, physical intervention may improve balance control for a particular patient even if it cannot totally reverse the balance impairment. Bradykinesia can be a composite effect of delayed alerting potentials, poor motor planning, rigidity (direct effects of the disease), and musculoskeletal limitations (indirect effects). Improvement of musculoskeletal flexibility might greatly improve a patient's ability to move quickly even though the alerting mechanism remains defective.

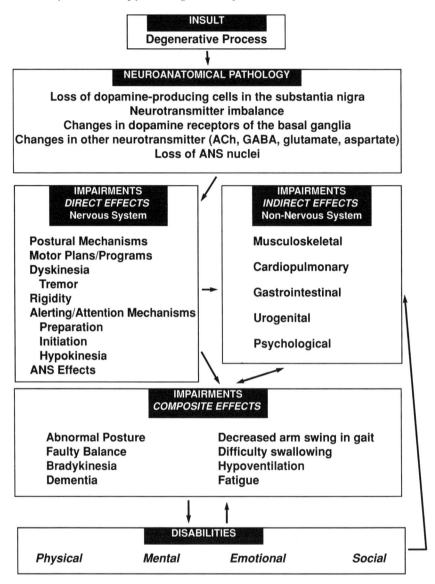

Fig. 9-5. The interrelationship of neuroanatomic pathology, impairments, and disabilities of PD. (Reprinted from Schenkman and Butler,[12] with permission.)

Schenkman and Butler[11,12] have outlined the relationship of disabilities, impairments, and neuroanatomic pathology in PD, illustrating the interrelationship of these phenomena (Fig. 9-5). The purpose of this analysis is to help clinicians focus on the causes of the PD patient's disability, and to then decide which impairments to attempt to correct, which to prevent, and when compensatory techniques should be used. The analysis should therefore facilitate the setting of appropriate goals, and should help the clinician decide which treatment strategies and techniques to use.

In the clinical setting of physical therapy, the purpose of an evaluation is to determine a patient's functional disabilities and to decide how best to remediate them. The interpretation of evaluation findings therefore begins with a patient's disabilities, to identify the patient's problems with function. The next step is to identify how impairments that are composite effects of the disease, such as those affecting balance, contribute to functional loss. Finally, the specific contributing impairments are identified. In other words, the model can be used to predict impairments and disability from pathology or to identify impairments from disability.

Application of the Analysis Technique

A case example best illustrates this approach to the analysis of disabilities in PD. This case has been chosen to demonstrate the thought process in interpreting a patient's disabilities. Complete, detailed, evaluative information is not presented, because the purpose of this case discussion is to illustrate the relationship between cause and effect. The specifics of the evaluation process are presented in the next section of this chapter.

FINDINGS
    The patient is a 67-year-old man with PD. He has been treated with alpha-methyldopa (Sinemet) for 3 years. At present, his status is

Disabilities

1. Physical

    Gait: Slow, lacks symmetrical coordination; (decreased extention throughout left lower extremity at heel strike and push off); decreased thoracolumbopelvic dissociation; wide base of support; takes 10 steps to complete a 360° turn.
    Sit-to-stand: Remains in a posterior pelvic tilt; rocks back and forth to start the activity; pushes up with hands; cannot rise from low surfaces.
    Bed mobility: Rolling and coming to sitting are slow an effortful; lacks trunk rotation and trunk lateral flexion during these activities.
    Speech: Quiet; difficult to hear.
    Writing: Small but accomplished without difficulty.
    Dressing: Sits to put on pants; some slowness in putting on shirt; lack of trunk flexibility during the task.
    Eating: Reports occasional tendency to drool.

2. Social

    States that he spends less time socializing than previously, owing to difficulties with speech and drooling. Stopped working 1 year ago.

3. Mental

Not formally assessed, but is alert, understands, and cooperates well with the evaluation. Appears to take initiative easily.

4. Emotional

States that he feels very isolated and discouraged.

Impairments

1. Composite Effects

Posture: Minimal thoracic kyphosis with significant forward head position more apparent during standing than sitting; slight left scoliosis; slight flexion of both left extremities when standing; posterior pelvic tilt when sitting.
Balance Control: Impaired sitting and standing:
Sitting: Cannot reach or shift weight to right side as well as to left; no automatic lower extremity movements when displaced to left by examiner.
Standing: Limited ability to maintain unilateral stance (left, 3 seconds; right, 10 seconds). No thoracolumbopelvic dissociation observed.
Bradykinesia
Rolling: Prone to supine (left or right): requires 10–14 seconds; sit-to-stand from treatment mat: 5 seconds.
Endurance: Complains of decreased tolerance for walking distances; fatigues during daily activities

2. Direct Effects

Rigidity: Moderate, left greater than right; affects trunk and neck as well as limbs.
Tremor: None apparent.
Reaction time: Not assessed as a separate entity.
Postural stability: No retropulsion noted; otherwise not assessed as a separate entity.
Planning/Programming: Does not appear to have difficulty in sequencing components of tasks, but was not formally assessed.

3. Indirect Effects

Range of motion: Tightness and lack of rotation and lateral flexion throughout spine, with greatest limitation in lumbopelvic area. Minimal selected decreases in range of motion of left extremities.
Respiration: Assessed by pulmonary function tests: within normal limits for age but at low end of normal.

INTERPRETATION

Slowness and awkwardness of movement appear to interfere greatly with all aspects of this individual's functional capacity and social and emotional status at the present time. In addition, drooling is becoming socially inhibiting for this patient. Rigidity combined with the resulting musculoskeletal limitations are probably the predominant causes of his physical disability. These impairments contribute to slowness in bed mobility and the rocking motion necessary to develop adequate momentum for moving from a sitting to standing position without the more appropriate trunk segmental movements. Balance impairments are also beginning to contribute to the patient's physical disability. This is apparent in his widened base of support and inability to perform a pivot turn. Rigidity combined with limitations of mobility are probably major contributors to the balance impairment. (Limitations in lumbopelvic mobility specifically, and trunk mobility generally, are contributors.) Balance impairments predispose this patient to future risk for falling and injury. Drooling may be a composite result of the excessive salivation associated with PD and the excessive forward head posture, which makes swallowing difficult. The forward head posture is in turn a result of rigidity. Respiratory function is not compromised at present, but is at risk for future impairment if loss of mobility progresses.

Intervention should be specifically directed at restoring mobility and postural alignment, with emphasis on the entire spine including the lumbopelvicfemoral area and the cervicothoracic area. As mobility increases, balance exercises should be initiated, with both self-initiated and externally initiated displacements emphasized. Preventive intervention should be initiated, including exercises for respiratory function and exercises requiring complex sequencing of motor tasks to maintain motor planning/programming skills. This patient has an apparent ability and motivation for participating in his care and for taking responsibility for long-term follow-through on exercises. In addition, his wife appears supportive and willing to assist him in any way necessary. This patient is therefore an excellent candidate for an intervention program that focuses on correction of his deficits and prevention of further impairments.

This patient should be reassessed on a regular basis to ensure that optimum posture and mobility are maintained and to reassess balance performance, motor planning/programming ability, and tremor. When these latter impairments progress to the point of interfering with functional capability, compensatory strategies should be initiated.

EVALUATION OF THE PARKINSON'S PATIENT

A comprehensive physical therapy evaluation is one of the keys to a successful intervention program for PD. Only when all of the patient's disabilities and impairments have been accurately assessed and interpreted can realistic goals and treatment strategies be identified. A comprehensive evaluation of the PD patient is particularly important in view of the complex and multi-faceted impairments that may contribute to the patient's disability from this disease.

In this section, evaluation techniques and approaches are reviewed for many of the disabilities and impairments of PD. This information is intended to serve three purposes for the clinician: (1) to provide guidance in structuring a comprehensive evaluation of the Parkinson's patient; (2) to summarize the interpretation of evaluation findings; and (3) to provide a basis for evaluation of PD patients for clinical studies of the efficacy of physical therapy intervention.

The components chosen for evaluation depend on how the information will be used. The first purpose of the evaluation is to determine the patient's functional capability. One consideration is to determine the patient's safety and the type of assistance needed. Another consideration in functional evaluation is to document a patient's status, in order to monitor the course of the disease and determine whether intervention is successful. When the findings of an evaluation are used for this purpose, it is necessary to document the patient's status using objective measures. The conditions of the evaluation must remain consistent, so that comparisons can be made over time. For the PD patient this means that the evaluation should always be done at a fixed time relative to the time when the patient takes antiparkinsonian medications. This is essential, given the great fluctuations in symptoms as the drugs are taken and as their effect wears off. It is also necessary for the evaluation procedures to be well enough specified so that the same or different evaluators can perform the assessment in a reproducible manner. The time it takes a patient to complete a functional task (such as transferring from bed to chair) is an example of an evaluation used for monitoring progress.

The second purpose of the evaluation is to interpret the cause of disability. The time taken to complete a task does not tell the therapist why the task is performed slowly or whether the task is performed in a mechanically appropriate fashion. Another consideration of the functional evaluation, is, therefore, to describe a particular activity, in order to interpret the reasons for a patient's dysfunction. For example, the description of how a patient transfers from the supine to the sitting position may help the therapist to interpret why the patient performs such a transfer slowly. Furthermore, the identification of such impairments as rigidity, limited mobility, or tremor may be useful in interpreting the causes of disabilities.

In general, a combination of descriptive and objective, quantifiable assessments is needed to describe comprehensively a patient's condition (Table 9-1).[8] Suggestions are given in this section for objective and descriptive assessments. The evaluation is presented in a stepwise fashion from disabilities to impairments, with differentiation between the various impairments in order to illustrate the thought process that occurs as evaluative information is obtained and interpreted. (This is not necessarily the ideal order for the actual evaluation in the clinic.)

Table 9-1. Examples of Problems, Interpretations, and Goals for Patients with Parkinson's Disease

Problem[a]	Quantitative	Descriptive	Interpretation	Goal
Gait	Ambulates 25 ft[b] in 18 sec (18 steps)	Small steps; decreased left heel-strike; decreased trunk rotation; left knee in flexion from weight acceptance to push-off; no left arm swing	Problems attributable to limitations in left knee and ankle range of motion and decreased available trunk rotation combined with trunk and limb rigidity with motor programming and planning deficits	Ambulate 25 ft in 10 sec (12 steps); improved heel-strike, push-off, trunk rotation, and arm swing
Bed mobility (supine to sitting)	7 sec to complete task	Lacks trunk rotation and dissociation of pelvic complex from shoulder complex; appears fearful of losing balance	Problems attributable to combination of limited available trunk range of motion, rigidity, and impaired balance	2 sec to complete task; improved trunk rotation with dissociation of shoulder complex from pelvic complex
Transfers (sitting to standing from low treatment table)	Sitting to standing from mat takes 10 sec	Lack of anterior pelvic tilt and of scooting forward on mat; excessive use of arms for push-off from mat	Problems attributable to lack of lumbopelvic mobility, rigidity, and difficulty motor planning and programming	Patient will accomplish task in 5 sec, use anterior tilt, scoot forward, and decrease need for use of arms
Decreased hip range of motion	Straight leg raise (left leg: 0°–50°; right leg: 0°–45°); internal rotation (left leg: 0°–25°; right leg: 0°–30°)		Problems result from rigidity and improper posturing	Hip range of motion within normal limits
Rigidity[c]		Moderate[d]	Attributable to primary impairments of disease	Patient will self-relax rigidity for increasing range of motion

[a] Patient problems may relate to disabilities or impairments.

[b] 1 ft = 0.3048 m.

[c] Rigidity is listed as a problem because of its causal role in most impairments of PD; however, objective measures of rigidity do not exist, and physical therapy does not appear to affect long-term changes.

[d] Feldman R, Lannon M: Parkinson's disease and related disturbances. p. 147. In Feldman R (ed): Neurology: The Physician's Guide. Thieme, New York, 1984.

(From Schenkman M, Donovan J, Tsubota J et al: Management of individuals with Parkinson's Disease: Rationale and Case Studies. Phys Ther 69:946, 1989, with permission.)

Overall Functional Status

An assessment of overall physical function can be useful in determining the PD patient's general level of capability. There are no available physical function evaluations for specific use with PD patients. However, the Functional Status Questionnaire[28] was developed to assess the ambulatory patients' level of difficulty with daily function. This questionnaire relies on the self-reporting of physical, psychological, and social function. The reliability of the subcomponents of the Functional Status Questionnaire has been established.[28] The Questionnaire or some similar scale can be used to screen and monitor the physical, psychological, and social function of the ambulatory PD patient.

Physical Disabilities: Gross Motor Skills

Typically, PD patients have difficulty with gross motor skills such as mobility in bed, coming to a standing from a sitting position, and gait. They may perform these tasks slowly and apparently with undue effort. Their trunk and neck appear stiff, with little rotational movement during function. It is therefore imperative to evaluate these functional activities early in the disease in order to identify and correct abnormalities of performance before they become functionally limiting.

Gross motor activities such as gait, mobility in bed, and transfer activities can be described from several perspectives: motion of body segments (i.e., kinematics), use of momentum, and stability characteristics (Tables 9-2 and 9-3). Kinematic descriptions of a task tell the reader how the individual body segments are used by a patient performing a task. In clinical evaluations, functional movements are generally described kinematically. Gait, for example, is frequently described in terms of the flexion and extension motions of the hip, knee, and ankle at heel strike, midstance, and push off. Trunk motion and arm swing are also described during gait.[29] Rolling for bed mobility can be described in terms of trunk motion (e.g., does the trunk rotate or is it held rigidly like a log?), whether the head and shoulders or the hips initiate the activity, and whether the arms are used to push or pull during rolling. Rising from the sitting to the standing position can be described in terms of the degree of the anterior or posterior pelvic tilt, how much the arms are used to push/pull the patient up, and whether the patient rocks back and forth to initiate the standing motion.

The kinematics of normal gait have been described by many authors,[30-32] and guidelines for the clinical assessment of gait are available.[33] With the exception of gait, there are only a few studies in the literature[34-36] that characterize the kinematics of gross motor tasks such as those described above. Such studies as do exist[34] serve to illustrate the broad range of kinematics used by healthy individuals performing gross motor activities. Without established guidelines for normal performance characteristics, the clinican relies on educated judgments and experience to decide whether a patient performs a particular gross motor activity in an appropriate manner.

Table 9-2. Examples of Kinematic, Momentum, Balance Control, and Timing Characteristics for Three Strategies of Standing Up from Sitting Down

Some Descriptors	Stability Strategy	Dynamic Strategy with Controlled Momentum Transfer	Uncontrolled Momentum Strategy
Kinematic	Pelvis in neutral alignment at initiation of task. Trunk is positioned in 45° of flexion before initiation of lift off. Upper extremities are used to push up from arm rests. Slight hip, knee, and ankle flexion at end of task.	Pelvis in neutral alignment at initiation of task. Rapid Trunk flexion before lift off of buttocks from chair seat. Forward flexion of trunk continues after lift off to about 30°. Upper extremities are not used for pushing. Full extension is achieved at end of task.	Pelvis in posterior tilt. Trunk is rapidly rocked forwards and backwards. Upper extremities are used to push up from arm rests. Patient takes several steps forward. Moderate flexion in trunk, hip, knee, and ankle at end of task.
Momentum	Momentum is not used in this strategy.	Trunk flexion velocity is used to generate momentum for the task and is transferred to generate vertical extension velocity as evidenced by the smooth continuous motion of the activity.	Rocking motion of the trunk is used to generate momentum to overcome posterior position of the body mass (owing to posterior pelvic tilt). Momentum is not transferred for vertical velocity but causes the patient to take several steps forward.
Balance control	Static stability mechanisms are used as evidenced by positioning of the upper body mass (trunk) over the feet before lift off.	Dynamic mechanisms are required because upper body mass (trunk) is positioned posteriorly relative to feet (new base of support) at the time of lift off of buttocks from chair seat.	Inherently unstable as evidenced by multiple steps to regain stability at end of task.
Timing from start to erect stance	2.5 seconds	1.3 seconds	4.0 seconds

Stability and momentum characteristics of functional movements can also help the clinician decide whether the patient performs a motor task appropriately.[16] Rising from the seated position can be used to illustrate this point. The seated person is inherently stable, with his or her body mass positioned directly over the seat. To stand up, the individual must shift body mass anteriorly and position the body over the feet, which serve as the new base of support. This can be accomplished using several strategies (Table 9-2). One strategy for

Table 9-3. Examples of Kinematic, Momentum, and Balance Control for Two Types of Gait

Some Descriptions	Dynamic Strategy	Stability Strategy
Kinematics	Hip, knee and ankle flexion appear within normal limits for gait. Lateral tilt of pelvis occurs as weight is transferred from one extremity to the other. Reciprocal arm swing occurs. Swing to stance ratio appears normal.	Shuffling steps with decreased hip, knee, and ankle flexion. No lateral tilt of pelvis observed as weight is transferred from one extremity to the other. No reciprocal arm swing observed. Increased period of double limb support.
Momentum	Momentum from forward progression of body is used. Eccentric action of lower extremity musculature controls forward progression.	Momentum strategy is not used. The requirement for eccentric control is minimized.
Balance control	Dynamic strategy is used.	Stability strategy is used as evidenced by increased double limb support time with transfer of body mass over stance limb before initiation of swing.

performing this activity relies on movement from one inherently stable position (sitting) to another (standing). For example, a person can flex the trunk far enough forward so that much of the body mass is already over the feet at the time when the buttocks leave a chair seat.[37] Alternatively, the individual can use a dynamic strategy that includes inherently unstable positions. For example, the person can develop momentum by moving the upper body quickly and rising from the seat while the body mass is still positioned more posteriorly (near the seat).[37] A third strategy, often seen in PD patients, is to rock the trunk back and forth to initiate the movement of rising. From the perspective of stability, this strategy is used when the pelvis remains tilted posteriorly during initiation of the sit-to-stand movement, forcing the patient to develop enough momentum to overcome the extreme posterior positioning of the body mass.

The first strategy described above for rising from a chair limits the period when the body mass is far from the base of support and therefore limits the period of dynamic stability. This strategy lessens the need for balance control. In the second example, the body mass is further from the base of support as the buttocks leave the chair seat. There is a greater period of dynamic stability, requiring considerable balance control when the buttocks leave the chair seat and until the body mass is securely positioned over the new base of support. The task must be accomplished more quickly using this strategy than when the first strategy is used. In the third example, considerable momentum is required to overcome the excessively stable posterior positioning of the body. The upper-body momentum is not transferred to the extension phase of the sit-to-stand activity but instead propels the body forward, necessitating stepping as stability is regained. In general, the strategy a patient uses for rising from sitting to standing balances the need for dynamic motion, the capacity for momentum generation, and the capability for momentum control. (Several recent studies provide examples of this type of kinetic analysis of the rising movement from sitting to standing, and interpret some of the reasons why patients might choose one strategy as opposed to another[36,37]). A description of stability and momentum characteristics can aid the clinician to interpret why a patient uses a particular kinematic strategy.

A similar approach can be used to analyze gait (Table 9-3). A person might walk quickly, allowing the swing extremity to leave the floor before body mass is positioned directly over the stance extremity. Alternatively, the person might not lift the swing extremity from the floor until the body mass is well positioned over the stance extremity. In this latter case, the gait would probably be slower and might appear as the "shuffling gait" frequently associated with PD. Reciprocal arm swing, with backward rotation of the thorax, provides a counterbalance to the forward rotation of the pelvis and lower extremity. If (as in PD) the thorax and pelvis do not rotate in opposite directions, then reciprocal arm swing would not be necessary and indeed would be kinetically inappropriate. The festinating gait associated with PD can also be interpreted from a kinetic perspective. It is possible that at least for some patients, the festinating gait occurs because the patient generates momentum and does not have adequate musculoskeletal flexibility to permit the balance control necessary to effectively modulate that momentum.

The description of the stability characteristics of a patient's functional movement, in combination with the kinematic characteristics, can help the clinician interpret why the patient moves as he or she does. From a combination of the kinematic and kinetic observations the clinician can begin to make educated deductions about mechanical constraints that dictate the patient's movement strategies. These deductions would be tested by further evaluation of the musculoskeletal system.

Observational assessments of functional movement do not provide a good means of monitoring a patient's status over time. Objective, reproducible assessments of functional movement are necessary for this purpose. Several authors have developed objective measures of physical function specifically for PD patients[7,9] and for elderly persons generally.[38] For example, the time it takes a patient to perform a task such as rolling over and coming to the sitting position can provide a useful measure of whether therapeutic intervention has helped the patient with bed mobility. Likewise, the time taken to rise from a chair and walk a set distance can help the therapist to monitor a patient's transfer capability. Both timing and step/stride characteristics can be used to objectively measure gait. For example, the time and number of steps can be measured as patients walk a set distance[7]; ink pads can be applied to the soles of the patient's shoes, followed by having the patient walk along a piece of brown paper. Step and stride characteristics can then be determined.[39] Most objective gait evaluations assess a person's gait when walking distances. This type of ambulation is normally done in a dynamic manner, with the COM outside the base of support most of the time.[40] In contrast, walking within the household is often a slower activity, with emphasis on shifting the COM slowly from one extremity to the other. Walking within the household is therefore less dynamic than distance walking. The reader can picture stepping and walking within the context of preparing dinner or washing dishes to visualize this type of gait activity. There are no objective, reliable assessments of this aspect of gait. The time and number of steps required to complete a 360° turn might provide a useful indication of a person's capability for this aspect of gait.

Physical Disabilities: Fine Motor Skills

Fine motor dysfunction can also become difficult early in PD. Impairments of fine motor function may make it difficult for the patient to perform such simple functional activities as buttoning a shirt or tying shoes. Disturbances in fine motor function can be evident in three areas: difficulty in initiating the task, slowness in completing the task, and difficulty in sequencing the various components necessary to complete the task. In addition, the capacity for eye–hand coordination, which is essential for many fine motor skills, may be impaired in PD patients, further compounding fine motor coordination. Descriptive evaluations of fine motor skills, such as buttoning clothes, writing, and eating, should be designed to differentiate between these aspects of a patient's disability. That is, the evaluation should describe apparent delays in initiating the movement, slowness in carrying out the movements needed for simple activities, and difficulty in simultaneously carrying out two different components of a task (e.g., stirring liquid while pouring other ingredients).

Few clinically applicable quantitative assessments of upper-extremity and fine motor skills are available specifically for PD patients. Wing et al.[41] have described tasks that can be used in the clinical setting, including a reciprocal arm-tapping task, the Purdue Pegboard for assessment of perceptual/motor coordination, and a line drawing task for assessment of reaction time. Palmer et al.[42] included a nine-hole pegboard test, a button board test, and a rapid alternating arm movement test as part of their evaluation battery in a study to assess the efficacy of intervention in PD. These and similar tests can be used to quantitate upper-extremity functional activitiy much as the time tasks described previously can be used to quantitate gross motor activities.

A number of investigators have attempted to further define the specific motor deficits of PD patients using tests of reaction time,[43] tracking tasks,[44–46] and repetitive movement tasks.[41] Although these tests require equipment beyond the scope of most clinical settings, they may be useful and appropriate for clinicians who wish to investigate experimentally the efficacy of intervention strategies in improving timing, tracking, or repetitive movement capability of PD patients.

In summary, a number of existing tests can be used to quantify gross and fine motor control specifically and functional ability in general. Some of the relevant tests have been summarized here. The clinician can choose from among the available tests according to the status of the patient to be evaluated. Furthermore, suggestions have been made for descriptive evaluations of functional movement that include characterization of both the components and the stability characteristics of such movement. While these evaluative tests describe and quantify function, they do not elucidate the causes of dysfunction. It is necessary to evaluate impairments in order to interpret the causes of any abnormalities of function identified by these assessments.

Impairments: Composite Effects of Parkinson's Disease

Impairments of posture and balance, as well as fatigue, can all be significant contributors to PD patients' disabilities in functional activities such as gait, mobility in bed, and rising from a sitting to a standing position. An important step in identifying the causes of disabilities in gross motor skills is therefore to determine whether posture, balance, or fatigue may be contributing factors. Each of these impairments may have multiple underlying causes, and are therefore considered composite effects of the disease. The identification of impairments of posture and balance as well as of fatigue will indicate that further evaluation is necessary to establish their underlying causes.

Posture

Impaired posture can potentially interfere with all gross motor activities because of the mechanical constraints that posture sets on movement. Typically, the posture of the PD patient becomes increasingly forward flexed and stooped.[1] Early in the disease, unilateral postural deviations may be observed in stance, including scoliosis and slight limb flexion on one side of the body. These are warning signs that musculoskeletal alterations are beginning to occur and should be treated. As the kyphosis and flexion increase, the position of the COM of the body is altered, and the patient's posture can interfere with all functions[16] (Figs. 9-2 and 9-6). Similarly, early in the disease, the PD patient may have a tendency to sit with a forward head and posterior pelvic tilt. This posture makes rising from a chair difficult and, unless corrected, may eventually lead to fixed musculoskeletal alterations.

The assessment of posture early in PD should therefore be done with attention to subtle postural alterations that are precursors to the postural deviations typical of the disease. Guidelines for postural evaluations in the standing position are available.[47] These guidelines should be modified to assess posture in the sitting as well as standing positions. Schenkman et al.[7] recommend the use of photographic records against a grid in order to assure better comparisons of posture over time. Figures 9-7 and 9-8 illustrate the use of photographs taken against a grid to demonstrate improvements in standing posture of a PD patient, following 6 weeks of physical intervention.

Objective measurement of postural deviations is more difficult. Webster[1] has recommended measuring how far anteriorly the head is positioned in relation to the most posterior aspect of the body. This measure gives a gross assessment

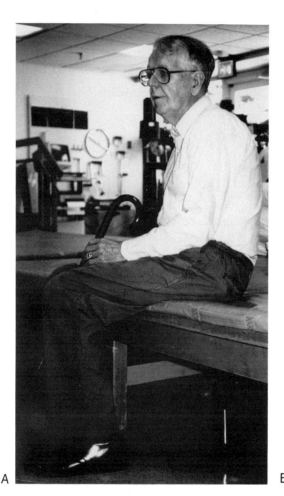
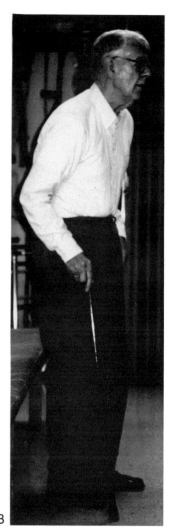

A   B

Fig. 9-6. Postural deviations observed early in Parkinson's disease. **(A)** Sitting posture illustrating the typical forward head and posterior pelvic tilt. **(B)** Standing posture of the same patient illustrating the similarity of head and pelvic positions.

of malalignment. Its reliability has not been established. Braun and Amundson[48] have recently developed an objective and reliable measure of the forward head position itself, which should be applicable and useful for the PD patient. The reliability of other postural assessments has not been reported.

There are a number of potential causes of postural abnormalities, including rigidity, bradykinesia, and musculoskeletal limitations. An interpretation of all evaluative findings may be necessary before the clinician can form educated hypotheses about the particular cause of postural abnormalities for a given patient.

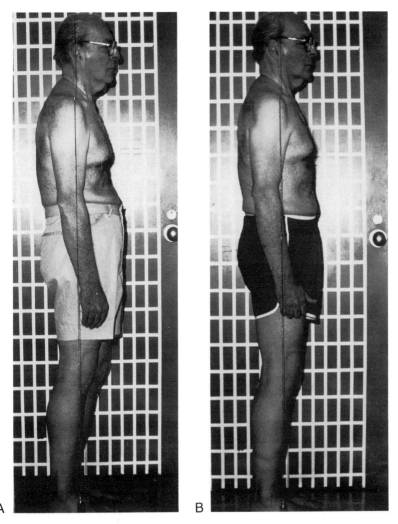

Fig. 9-7. Use of photographs taken against a grid to document postural changes. **(A)** Lateral view before physical therapy intervention. **(B)** Lateral view following 6 weeks of physical therapy intervention.

Balance

Balance impairment or a disorder of postural stability is one of the hallmarks of PD.[2,3,9] Impaired balance can interfere with all functional activities and can lead to serious injury and further disability. In fact, falls are a common accompaniment of the disease as it progresses, often leading to hip fracture,[49,50] which can in turn lead to death.[51] Balance control is required for patients to use strategies of movement that require dynamic stability. A strategy of movement that positions the COM away from the center of force (COF), requires a degree of balance control that is adequate to maintain stability. For example, when

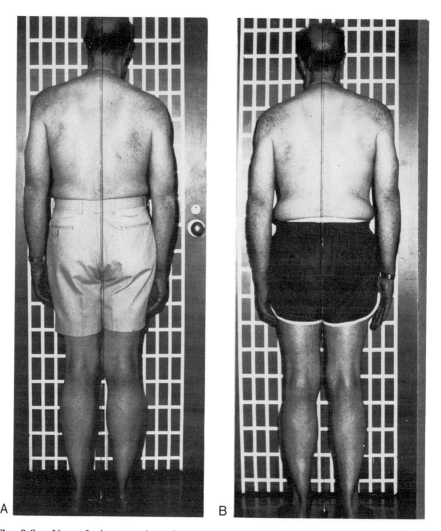

Fig. 9-8. Use of photographs taken against a grid to document postural changes. **(A)** Posterior view before physical therapy intervention. **(B)** Posterior view following 6 weeks of physical therapy intervention.

rising from the sitting to the standing position, an individual can lift the buttocks from the chair seat before the COM is positioned directly over the COF of the feet.[36,37] When this strategy is used, the COM and COF are relatively far apart. Under static conditions the body mass would pull the person down posteriorly. This strategy of rising from a chair requires dynamic control so that the person does not fall back into the seat. The strategy also requires dynamic control to ensure that the COM does not progress too far anteriorly during forward movement, causing the person to fall forward. Without adequate balance control, a PD patient might rely on a less dynamic strategy, such as positioning the trunk well forward over the feet and then pushing upward to the standing position.[37]

Gait similarly requires balance control. Normally the COM deviates considerably from the COF during gait, so that the walking person is constantly controlling the limits of his or her COM to prevent instability and falling.[40] Without adequate balance control, step length may be shortened, the base of support widened, and the COM moved over the new support limb prior to toe-off at all times. Such a strategy of movement eliminates the typical dynamic stability of gait.

Simple functional tasks, such as reaching forward to pick up a jar from a shelf or bending down to tie one's shoes, likewise require dynamic stability and balance control. In short, dynamic stability is requried throughout the day, and balance control is essential for that stability. Finally, balance control is also required in response to external perturbations, such as those experienced when a person is jostled in a crowd, trips over a scatter rug, or walks on an uneven surface.

Balance control should be assessed both for self-initiated displacements of COM and in response to external perturbations. A growing number of investigators have begun to develop assessments of balance control that are useful for both purposes. As with assessments of functional movement, some of these evaluations yield objective data, others yield descriptive information; the evaluator must decide which measurements to use.

There are various possible causes for impaired balance in PD, including both direct and indirect effects of the disease. Evidence suggests that for some PD patients, impaired balance may be due to a deficit in the preparatory postural responses that normally occur prior to voluntary movement.[52,53] There may also be abnormalities of the postural stretch reflexes[54-56] and inability to coordinate postural responses with voluntary movement.[53,57,58]

It has also been suggested that musculoskeletal limitations contribute directly to impaired postural responses to PD patients.[7,16] From a purely mechanical perspective, loss of mobility of the lumbopelvofemoral area or of the cervical area puts structural limits on a patient's capacity for a normal balance response.[16] Furthermore, the flexed and stiff parkinsonian posture, with forward head and thoracic kyphosis, necessarily alters the normal effects of gravity acting on the body, and hence should influence postural response mechanisms. The relationship between mechanical limitations and the PD patient's impaired balance has not received adequate attention and deserves experimental study for several reasons. First and foremost, musculoskeletal limitations are perhaps the most responsive of all of the PD patient's impairments to physical therapeutic techniques. There is good reason to expect improvement of balance if musculoskeletal impairments are a significant contributing factor to imbalance. Second, musculoskeletal impairments make it difficult to definitively identify abnormalities of postural response mechanisms, because the mechanical limitations they impose can mask the impairment of the postural response mechanism itself.

When evaluating balance (as when evaluating functional movement), the therapist should decide which purposes the balance assessment should serve (e.g., to ascertain safety, to describe the outcome of a balance response, or to

Table 9-4. Balance Assessments for Different Purposes

Safety	Describe the level of assistance required under a variety of conditions.
Components of the Balance Response[16,60,61]	
self initiated perturbations	Use perturbations such as reaching, shifting COM from one side of the pelvis to the other, and unilateral stance. Describe head, trunk, neck, and limb adjustments of position.
external perturbations	Use perturbations such as tilting the patient with force applied at the pelvis in sitting and standing. Describe head, trunk, neck, and limb adjustments of position.
Documentation of Progress[16,62–64]	Use time and force plate measures to quantify variables such as the time the patient can maintain a posture (such as unilateral stance) or the distance the patient can move COM away from a central point.

monitor progress). Balance control should be evaluated in response to both self-initiated and external perturbations. To illustrate this point, a few assessments are summarized in Table 9-4. Tinetti[38] has developed an assessment of balance control within functional activities such as rising from a chair, twisting, reaching, bending down, and walking. Performance on this evaluation scale has been shown to relate to the probability of falling.[59]

A number of authors[60,61] have described the components of the balance response that might be expected when PD patients are tested in the sitting or standing position. These evaluations describe limb, neck, and trunk responses. Schenkman[16] has suggested linking the observed kinematic responses to specific spinal motions in order to adequately characterize the musculoskeletal response.

Balance can also be quantitated in order to monitor progress. Performance can be quantitated using very simple measures (e.g., how long a patient maintains a unilateral stance)[16,62] or more sophisticated measures (e.g., alteration of the COM in relation to the center of pressure [COP] as measured by force platforms.[63,64]). The conditions under which balance control is tested can also be varied by manipulation of the support surface, visual environment, or type of perturbation.[62]

However one decides to test balance control, the interpretation of the assessment results is critical because it will directly influence the choice of an intervention strategy. First, the findings should be interpreted with respect to patient safety. The patient at risk for falls or injury should be taught compensatory strategies of movement to prevent injury, at least until such time as his or her balance control improves. Second, it is important to determine the circumstances under which balance is most impaired. Are the patient's balance responses worse when the patient is externally perturbed or when the patient alters his or her COM/COP relationship through self-initiated movement? Third, it is necessary to interpret how the balance impairment affects functional movement. Do the patient's gait or transfer strategies reflect an attempt to limit dynamic stability because of poor balance control? Finally, it is necessary to consider the balance-assessment findings within the context of the overall evaluative findings to reach an educated clinical hypothesis about the major factors contributing to a patient's balance impairment (Fig 9-3). In particular, it is important to decide whether musculoskeletal limitations play a major role in decreased balance control, whether there appear to be abnormalities in the postural response system itself, and whether rigidity, bradykinesia, or poor motor planning/programming might be contributory. There is no foolproof method for making such a clinical hypothesis; rather the clinician must rely on previous experience and clinical skill, and then confirm or reject the hypothesis based on the patient's response to intervention.

Endurance

Decreased endurance and fatigue of the PD patient has been referred to in the literature, but has not been well characterized.[65] Various impairments could contribute to decreased endurance in PD, including loss of skeletal muscle, cardiopulmonary impairments, the effort of constantly moving against the resistance of rigidity and bradykinesia, and depression.[12,65] Standard evaluations of cardiopulmonary endurance can and should be used to evaluate and monitor this important impairment. The evaluation of general musculoskeletal endurance has not been well delineated, although the endurance of specific muscle groups can be established with Cybex or similar testing.

Drooling

Drooling is one of the socially disabling aspects of PD, and is associated with the excessive salivation produced by the dysfunctional autonomic nervous system in the disease.[12] It has been suggested that the forward head position in PD may contribute to this impairment by making it difficult for the patient to swallow.[12] Although this suggestion has not yet been investigated, it would seem logical that an improved head position should improve swallowing and therefore lessen the drooling. Since musculoskeletal impairments contributing to the forward head position might be prevented or retarded through physical therapy techniques, these contributions to drooling should be carefully considered.

In summary, postural abnormalities, balance dysfunction, decreased endurance, and drooling can each contribute significantly to the PD patient's total disability. It is important to establish the presence of these impairments and to interpret their possible contribution to the patient's disabilities. Once impairments of posture, balance, endurance, and drooling have been identified, further evaluation is necessary to understand their underlying causes. These impairments must be interpreted in the light of evaluative findings about the impairments of a patient's neurologic system (e.g., rigidity, tremor, planning/programming), musculoskeletal system, and cardiopulmonary system.

Impairments: Direct Effects of Parkinson's Disease

The following impairments can arise from the neuroanatomic pathology of PD: rigidity, tremor, postural instability, akinesia, and impairments of motor planning and programming. Some of these impairments are difficult to evaluate as isolated phenomena; others are difficult to quantitate using clinically applicable techniques. It is nevertheless important for the clinician to attempt to assess the extent to which these impairments occur as a direct effect of the disease and to interpret their contribution to the patient's total disability. Each of these impairments will be discussed in terms of its probable cause and its role in producing disability in PD; evaluation of each will be summarized.

Rigidity

Rigidity in PD has been attributed to a failure of relaxation of the voluntary motor system.[27,66] That is, the muscles of patients with parkinsonian rigidity are in a constant and excessive state of alertness. Rogers[55] has recently summarized the potential neurophysiologic sources and correlates of rigidity, which include an increased tonic resting state of muscles or an increased responsiveness to passive stretch. The long-latency electromyographic response to stretch during movement appears to be abnormal in rigidity. Cogwheeling is frequently observed and has been interpreted as a combination of rigidity and tremor. Rigidity is known to increase with stress or anxiety[55] as well as with effort.

The role of rigidity in producing motor dysfunction and functional disability in PD is controversial. The work of Dietz and colleagues suggests that the abnormal neurophysiologic responses of patients who exhibit rigidity may interfere with their control of stance and gait.[54] Berger et al. have suggested that rigidity contributes to the flexed parkinsonian posture.[67] In addition, rigidity has been implicated as a contributor to the respiratory impairments of PD patients.[9,68] Clinical experience strongly supports the role of rigidity in producing musculoskeletal limitations.[1,7] The clinician must make educated judgments about the role of rigidity in contributing to a particular patient's impairments and to altered functional mobility. These judgments should be based on an analysis of all evaluative findings.

Approaches to the evaluation and quantitation of rigidity have varied from the use of clinically feasible scoring systems to sophisticated electromyographic or force scoring systems. Scales that rate the severity of rigidity from none present to severe, based on resistance to passive movement, have been used by both clinicians and researchers.[9,69] Feldman and Lannon[9] include the effect of reinforcement or effort on rigidity by assessing the rigidity of the opposite extremity while the patient makes a fist. They consider fixed postural defects as evidence of severe rigidity. Generally, these tests score rigidity of the extremities but not the trunk. This is an oversight that should be corrected. Identification of rigidity of the trunk may help the clinician establish the link between rigidity, altered postural alignment, and eventual loss of mobility throughout the trunk.

The clinical scoring systems described above do not provide reliable values of rigidity,[70] especially when used to assess persons who have mild rigidity.[69] Nevertheless, it is important for the clinician to consider the possible contribution of rigidity to a patient's total disability, and it is therefore necessary to use some system of scoring rigidity clinically even if the results are not ideal.

A number of investigators have developed more sophisticated and objective measures of rigidity of the extremities, including the Wartenberg pendulum test,[71] which measures relaxation time after the limb is dropped; of a hanging limb[73]; and resistance torque during forearm flexion and extension,[42] a measurement of net work when the forearm is flexed and extended through a 100° arc at constant velocity.[73] These tests may be useful in studies designed to investigate the relationship between rigidity and specific aspects of dysfunction. They are also appropriate for studies designed to investigate whether physical therapy intervention alters rigidity in PD patients.

Tremor

Tremor affects almost all patients with PD,[2] and when moderate or severe can interfere significantly with fine motor control.[9] Tremor can be characterized either qualitatively or quantitatively. Some authors rate tremor subjectively (none, minimal, moderate, severe)[74] or measure tremor in terms of its frequency in cycles per second,[45] its amplitude, or both.[58] Palmer et al.[42] characterized tremor in terms of elbow torque generated during a mental activation task. Feldman and Lannon[9] developed a five-point scale that scores tremor on the basis of whether it occurs at rest or with movement, and estimates the extent to which tremor interferes with function. Fahn and colleagues[75] have developed a much more comprehensive assessment of tremor using a five-point scale. They rate tremor of the head, face, trunk, and extremities at rest and in maintained postures. They also rate tremor during functional activities including writing, speaking, feeding, and hygiene.

Bradykinesia

Bradykinesia has long been considered one of the cardinal signs of PD,[2,3,76] and has been attributed directly to CNS dysfunction associated with the disease. It is increasingly evident that the bradykinesia in PD does not result from a single abnormality. At the neurophysiologic level it has at least two broad causes: a delay in the time required to initiate a movement (probably correlated with a delay in alerting mechanisms),[76] and an increase in the time to execute the movement.[55] There is some suggestion that the increased time taken for executing a movement is partly due to a differential impairment of ramp as compared to ballistic mechanisms for motor output.[5,76] Other factors that may contribute to a PD patient's overall difficulty in moving in a timely fashion include difficulty with motor planning/programming for complex motor acts, lack of adequate postural stability for controlling movement when using strategies requring dynamic stability, and loss of the musculoskeletal flexibility needed for segmental movement. In the clinical setting it may be impossible to differentiate between motor control deficits of a particular patient for initiation as opposed to execution of movements. An evaluative finding of slowness of movement should therefore be interpreted in conjunction with findings related to postural stability, motor plans/programs, and musculoskeletal flexibility. With this in mind, the tests previously described for fine and gross motor control can be interpreted with respect to a primary slowness in initiating or executing movements.

Postural Instability

Postural instability is another impairment that can result from a specific abnormality of the postural response mechanisms. However, postural instability may be compounded by delayed reaction time, rigidity, or musculoskeletal limitations. Clinically, it may be impossible to evaluate a primary impairment of postural instability in isolation from other factors that can interfere with balance. Tests of postural stability are therefore discussed under the broad category of balance, along with other composite effects of PD, and without an attempt to use clinical tests to isolate the component that is a direct effect of the disease.

Motor Planning/Programming

Impairments of motor planning/programming have long been associated with PD, although the terminology *plan/program* has only been well articulated in the past decade.[5,27,77,78] In 1964, Schwab observed that PD patients have an inability to perform two motor acts simultaneously.[70] Marsden[5] characterized this difficulty as an inability to simultaneously run two different motor programs in order to execute a complex motor plan. He described the difficulties of a PD patient in simultaneously standing up from a chair and shaking someone's hand. Either the patient succeeded in rising from the chair as his outstretched hand dropped to his side, or managed to keep the hand outstretched for a handshake but fell back into the chair. The "freezing" phenomenon characteristic of PD may be another example of impaired planning/programming capability. A patient may successfully walk down a hallway until encountering an unexpected obstacle in his or her path. At this point the patient may falter or freeze from inability to plan a strategy to circumvent the obstacle while simultaneously planning for gait.

This difficulty in the simultaneous execution of different motor programs can, if severe, be quite disabling. It is important for the clinician to identify the impairment and to develop strategies that will help the patient compensate for the impairment. A few evaluative tests have been described that can help the clinician assess this impairment.[45,70] Talland and Schwab[70] described two manual tasks that can be performed in any clinic setting. In the first test, the patient holds a tally counter in the nondominant hand and presses it repeatedly and as fast as possible. At the same time, he or she uses the dominant hand to transfer beads from one bowl to another. The scoring in this test is based on the number of beads transferred in a set time, as compared to the score achieved by control subjects without PD.

The second test described by Talland and Schwab[70] is a crossing-out task in which both hands are used, depending on the location on a page of the letters that are to be crossed out. Patients with PD performed this task more slowly with either hand than did control subjects, as anticipated by the investigators. The gap between the PD patients and controls widened, however, when the task became bimanual, thus supporting the use of this task to evaluate deficits in the simultaneous use of different motor programs.

Flowers[45] developed a slightly more sophisticated task, which involved step-tracking designed to differentiate between the initial impulse for a motor act and secondary adjustments. Sharpe et al.[78] have described a gestural test that was also designed to identify deficits in planning.

In summary, such direct effects of PD as rigidity, decreased reaction time, increased performance time, and deficits in motor planning/programming can all significantly interfere with movement and functional ability. Clinical evaluations of bradykinesia, motor planning/programming, and postural instability have not been refined to the point at which it is possible to definitively differentiate between these impairments as sources of motor dysfunction and functional disability. The available clinical tests for timing and coordination of fine motor activities, for example, may not be selective enough to permit a definitive differentiation between rigidity, decreased reaction time, increased performance time, and deficits in motor planning/programming as causative impairments. Yet the strategy for intervention may differ significantly according to the specific causes of an impairment. Intervention for bradykinesia due predominantly to a decreased reaction time or increased performance time may require the practice of specific tasks at progressively increasing speeds; intervention for bradykinesia due to difficulties of motor planning for use of sequential motor programs may entail practicing increasingly complex sequential tasks, and may ultimately require compensatory techniques such as conscious sequencing strategies; intervention for bradykinesia due to loss of flexibility would include techniques for increasing range of motion and flexibility. It is therefore essential for the evaluator to form the best possible clinical hypothesis of how the impairments described above contribute to a patient's functional disability before selecting an optimum treatment strategy for the patient.

Furthermore, physical interventions cannot remediate impairments that result directly from neuroanatomic pathology of PD. These impairments, by definition, result from the loss of neuroanatomic structures and resulting neurophysiologic abnormalities. They are the impairments most likely to respond positively to pharmacologic intervention.[12] It is important in setting goals related to physical therapeutic intervention in PD to decide whether impairments are most likely to respond to physical or pharmacologic intervention, and to decide whether physical therapeutic techniques should be directed at correcting an impairment, compensating for it, or preventing other impairments. Although it is impossible to definitively determine the percentage of a specific impairment, such as bradykinesia, that results directly from the disease, it is important and necessary for the clinician to form an educated clinical hypothesis about this based on an interpretation of all the evaluative findings for a particular patient. Furthermore the patient's response to pharmacologic intervention provides important evidence about whether an impairment is a direct effect of the disease. If the impairment improves at the time that antiparkinsonian medications are taken, and worsens as the medications wear off, then the impairment is presumed to be directly caused by the disease. The careful use of objective measures of impairments is necessary to make this determination. If an impairment is unaffected by antiparkinsonian medication, the several possible explanations for this include the possibility that the impairment is an indirect effect of the disease, that it has both direct and indirect contributions, or that it is a direct effect of the disease but is unaffected by the medication chosen.

Impairments: Indirect Effects of Parkinson's Disease

Musculoskeletal impairments are perhaps the most important of all indirect effects of PD for the physical therapist to evaluate and treat. These impairments may interfere with balance, all functional movements, respiratory function, and endurance. Musculoskeletal impairments may also contribute to the upper-extremity pain that PD patients frequently report. This section of the evaluation therefore includes assessment of the patient's musculoskeletal system, respiratory system, and of pain.

Musculoskeletal Evaluations

Musculoskeletal evaluations have been described by many authors,[47,79–82] and will not be reviewed in detail here. The components of the musculoskeletal evaluation should include range of motion, strength, and muscle endurance. Evaluation of range of motion must include the trunk and neck, since these areas are often affected early in the disease, and loss of trunk/neck mobility has a profound mechanical effect on movement,[16] potentially interfering with balance responses and making rolling and coming to a standing position difficult. While objective measures of limb range of motion have been well described, objective

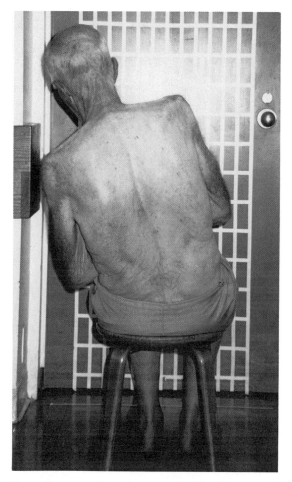

Fig. 9-9. Available trunk range of motion recorded by photographic record with the patient in front of a grid. (From Schenkman M,[16] with permission.)

measures for documenting trunk and neck motion have only recently become available.[48,81,82] A photographic record of the patient, taken against a grid, can be used to provide a permanent qualitative record of available motion (Fig. 9-9). The therapist should determine which of the patient's functional movements would be most affected by each restriction. Thus, for example, loss of cervical mobility interferes with driving, while loss of lumbopelvic mobility impairs weight shifting in while standing.

Range-of-motion assessments should differentiate between loss of range due to soft-tissue limitations and loss of range due to articular changes. Techniques of joint mobilization can be used for this purpose. It is also necessary to attempt to differentiate between those limitations of motion that result from PD and those that occur in elderly individuals as a result of the many other conditions and diseases affecting this age group. (Such differentiation will help to guide the clinician in terms of aggresssiveness of intervention and probable success in restoring mobility).

Although there are some suggestions that strength and/or endurance may be limited in PD patients,[65] the link between these impairments and the disease is not well established. Nevertheless, it is important for the clinician to establish the patient's capability and limitations in these areas, again hypothesizing about whether a particular impairment is directly or indirectly due to PD or is related to other aspects of aging. Standard protocols for measuring muscle strength are available.[47] Muscle endurance, typically measured with the Cybex™ or related equipment, has not been reported for PD patients, although such studies would be of value in identifying impairments of their endurance. If strength or endurance is diminished, it is necessary to interpret the extent to which these impairments limit a patient's functional movement and the extent to which they could be improved through appropriate exercise.

Respiratory Impairments

Respiratory impairments are clearly a common accompaniment to PD.[4] There is some suggestion in the literature that these impairments may partly result from an obstructive ventilatory deficit caused by the extrapyramidal deficits in motor control in PD.[4,83,84] Respiratory dysfunction could also be attributed to the restrictive effects of the kyphotic posture in PD. This latter impairment may be preventable through an intervention designed to delay or prevent postural and musculoskeletal abnormalities. It is therefore important to monitor a patient's respiratory status beginning early in the disease. Standard pulmonary function tests of vital capacity, forced expiratory volume, flow rate, and other parameters can be used for this purpose. If the clinician does not have access to equipment for pulmonary function tests, he or she should at least record the patient's inspiratory-to-expiratory ratio during breathing, and should describe the chest and the apparent pattern of breathing.

Pain

Pain is frequently described by PD patients, and is often noted with shoulder movement. Pain should be noted and the clinician should then perform a careful musculoskeletal evaluation to determine whether it has specific musculoskeletal causes. For example, the shoulder bursitis that frequently accompanies PD may be caused by a patient's kyphotic thoracic posturing, with resulting scapular malalignment coupled with weakness of the lower trapezius muscles.

Dystonic Movements

Dystonic movements often occur in PD patients as a side effect of antiparkinsonian medications.[9] These movements wax and wane as the effects of the medications wax and wane. They should be documented and their interference with functional movement interpreted.

In summary, PD can lead indirectly to impairments in musculoskeletal and respiratory function and to pain, all of which can significantly contribute to a patient's total disability. These impairments can be delayed by appropriate physical therapeutic management, and can be reversed, at least to some extent, if treated early in the disease.[7,12] It is therefore important to identify these impairments early in the disease, to interpret their role in a patient's altered posture, balance, and endurance, and to direct treatment toward the musculoskeletal and respiratory systems when appropriate. Perhaps the greatest efficacy of physical therapeutic techniques in PD is in managing these indirect effects of the disease. Their role in disability, and the importance of remediation, cannot be overemphasized.

SETTING GOALS

Once the evaluation findings are complete and have been interpreted in relation to each other, the clinician is ready to set goals for treatment. The broad goal of treatment is to preserve independent function for as long as possible. This is accomplished by addressing underlying impairments. The goals of physical therapy may therefore relate to both function and impairments.

Several factors should be considered when setting goals. First it is important to determine the patient's own goals and to decide who realistically will be most responsible for the long-term continuation of physical therapy: the patient, family members, or other caregivers. This will help in deciding whether the correction of various impairments is realistic and warranted. For example, it may not be useful to correct loss of trunk and neck mobility in a physical therapy program unless the exercises so used will be continued at home to preserve the gains that are made in mobility.

Second, it is necessary to decide which impairments should be corrected and which prevented, and those for which compensation should be made. Goals can then be clearly stated and can be realistically based on motor control, musculoskeletal, and cardiopulmonary dysfunction. The therapist may, for example, propose to correct losses of musculoskeletal flexibility and posture, to prevent recurrence of pneumonia, and to compensate for tremor. The decision about correction, compensation, and prevention is determined by factors such as whether the impairment is a direct effect of PD, how pre-existing medical conditions or the normal effects of aging contribute to a problem, and the patient's capability for long-term, self-directed exercise.

Third, it is important to articulate goals in quantitative terms, so that the success of the intervention program can be monitored. Particularly with PD, which is chronic and progressive, it is important to objectively document the patient's status. It is easy to miss changes (whether progressive or regressive) when goals are described vaguely.

In summary, the goals of a physical therapeutic program for PD should be realistically determined by underlying impairments, should be appropriate for the patient's own goals, needs, and home environment, and should be measurable. Table 9-1 outlines a few problems associated with PD, their interpretation, and goals in treating them.

TREATMENT FOR THE AMBULATORY PARKINSON'S PATIENT

General Approach

The treatment strategies and techniques outlined in this section are designed to address the motor-control dysfunction in PD through a mechanically and kinesiologically sound approach.[7] Rigidity and bradykinesia can be considered motor-control impairments that lead indirectly to many of the musculoskeletal and respiratory impairments of PD. The approach to physical therapy intervention in PD therefore centers around reduction of rigidity and the use of regular, appropriate, and frequent movement to circumvent these indirect effects on the musculoskeletal and respiratory systems.

A mechanical and kinesiologic analysis of the PD patient's posture and movement indicates that proximal musculoskeletal impairments are major contributors to functional disability. Musculature and joint mobility in the neck and vertebral column can be severely compromised even early in the disease. From a mechanical and kinesiologic perspective, treatment therefore begins while the patient is in supported, mechanically less demanding postures, with emphasis on the trunk musculature and intervertebral mobility. The initial purposes of therapy are to restore more normal alignment, mobility, and flexibility of the neck and trunk so that the patient will have a more normal basis for optimum limb function. The long-term goals of therapy are to prevent musculoskeletal limitations that contribute to impairments of respiratory and balance control and to physical dysfunction.

The breakdown in motor planning and programming that has been associated with PD[5,27] dictates that physical therapy for the disease should specifically incorporate the repetitive practice of functional activities that require simultaneous sequencing of different motor programs. The sequences chosen should be simple and easy to remember. The deficits in the postural response mechanism that result directly from the disease suggest that the practice of complex motor acts should include activities that require balance control. It is important for the patient to preserve for as long as possible the ability to integrate automatic postural responses with movement that is controlled consciously. These aspects of the treatment approach reflect a belief that PD patients may have a capability for improved coordination of conscious and automatic motor behavior, but may require repetitive practice to retain and optimize all of these motor routines as the disease progresses.

The motor control impairment that results in the tremor of PD is not generally considered responsive to physical therapeutic interventions, although Palmer et al.[42] do report its improvement with such therapy. If tremor interferes with function, compensatory strategies should be explored with the patient in order to maximize the patient's capability for effective use of the upper extremities. The dystonic behavior often associated with pharmacologic intervention in PD[9] may likewise not respond to physical therapeutic intervention. Compensatory strategies and patient awareness, as well as consultation with the primary physician or neurologist about the possible reduction of side effects through changes in medication or dosage, are similarly indicated for this impairment.

All interventional strategies and exercises for the PD patient can and should be made functionally relevant. A kinesiologic and mechanical structuring of intervention does not and should not preclude its functional relevance. There is, in fact, a growing awareness of the need for treatment regimens to be grounded in functionally meaningful contexts and to be goal-directed.[85] Practical experience also supports the notion that PD patients are most likely to comply with exercises on an ongoing basis if they find functional meaning in the exercises and find that the exercises lead to improvement in their daily functional capacity.

Finally, PD is a progressive, chronic disorder. The most important aspect of beneficial intervention for its management is therefore patient and family teaching. Ultimately, the patient and/or the patient's family must be able to assume responsibility for ongoing compliance with a home program for managing the disease if interventional strategies for its management are to be of lasting benefit for the patient.

Suggested Progression of Exercises

This section outlines a progression of exercises that is derived from the preceding philosophy.[7,12] The progression is intended to be used over time (across treatment sessions), and is also intended as a structure to be used within individual treatment sessions. This strategy assumes limitations of mobility throughout the patient's spine and extremities. The techniques described can be modified to address only the relevant areas if musculoskeletal limitations are confined to certain areas of the patient's body.

Relaxation of Excessive Muscle Tension

Relaxation of excessive muscle tension is one of the keys to all other interventional strategies in PD, and should therefore be addressed first. Muscle tension from rigidity should be reduced prior to range-of-motion exercises, balance activities, or practice of functional activities. The first task in physical therapy intervention is to teach techniques of muscle relaxation. These techniques can be most effective if the patient learns self relaxation to counteract rigidity. This assumes that the patient has an adequate level of attention and self direction. If the patient is not capable of carrying through with self-relaxation techniques, it may be possible to teach family members or other caregivers to assist the patient with muscle relaxation techniques.

Breathing Exercises

Breathing exercises are also employed early in the intervention in PD, for two reasons. First, they can aid in relaxation[86] and should therefore be taught in conjunction with relaxation techniques. Second, respiratory complications occur frequently in PD. In fact, pneumonia is one of the leading causes of death of PD patients.[2] It is therefore important to teach appropriate breathing exercises early in the disease in order to have the patient retain maximal respiratory capability and to prevent untimely loss of vital capacity and compromised ability to clear secretions.

Range-of-Motion and Flexibility Exercises

Range-of-motion and flexibility exercises are the third aspect of treatment to be emphasized early in PD. Adequate range of motion and flexibility are mechanical necessities if the patient is to perform functional activities in an optimal manner. Range of motion and flexibility within each segment of the vertebral column are at least as important as are range of motion and flexibility of limb segments. Full range of motion of the extremities probably cannot be optimally utilized for function unless there is full mobility of more proximal structures as well. For example, a fully mobile wrist and elbow can be optimally utilized only if the patient's glenohumeral motion is within normal limits. Glenohumeral motion will be restricted if scapular motion is restricted. Scapular motion will in turn be restricted if the thorax is excessively kyphotic, positioning the scapula abnormally. The approach to increasing flexibility and range of motion therefore begins with the trunk and proceeds to the extremities.

Active-Movement Exercises

Active-movement exercises serve two purposes. They can assist in restoration of range of motion and flexibility. They are also necessary for the restoration of more effective coordination of motor control for functional activities. Coordination of motor performance requires appropriate sequencing of conscious repertoires of movement in conjunction with appropriate automatic programs of movement. Thus, active-movement exercises should include both conscious and automatic repertoires. Automatic repertoires that relate to balance control during functional activities occur both in response to self-initited displacement of the COM and in response to externally initiated disturbances of the COM. It is important to practice both types of automatic repertoires.

Specific Treatment Techniques

Fully Supported Positions

Relaxation techniques in PD are specifically directed at reducing excessive muscle tension due to rigidity.[7] The exact mechanism underlying the rigidity in PD has not yet been well established. It appears, however, that rigidity occurs

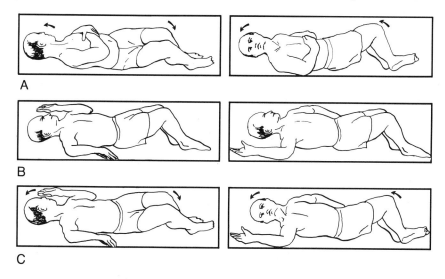

Fig. 9-10. Sequence of exercises that can be used in supine to increase range of motion of the neck and trunk. Any combination of motions can be used. **(A)** Head is slowly rotated side to side within the available range of motion while lower extremities are rotated side to side *in the opposite direction*. **(B)** Upper extremities are positioned in 45 degrees of shoulder abduction with 90 degrees of elbow flexion. One shoulder is externally rotated; the opposite shoulder is internally rotated. From this initial position the shoulders are slowly rotated back and forth from an internally to an externally rotated position. **(C)** In an advanced exercise the head, shoulders, and lower extremities are simultaneously rotated from one position to the other.

because muscles are cortically or subcortically activated in the absence of specific peripheral sensory stimuli.[27,66] Techniques for reducing rigidity should therefore reflect an attempt to centrally turn down the level of muscle activation. Slow rotational motions through small ranges of motion have reportedly been effective in temporarily reducing rigidity.[7] These rotational motions can be performed by the patient, by the therapist assisting the patient, or both.

Following the kinesiologic model, relaxation exercises should be initiated with the patient in a fully supported position (e.g., supine or side-lying). In the supine position it is possible to relax the muscles of the neck by slow, side-to-side rotational movements of the head (Fig. 9-10). It is possible to relax muscles of the low back area by side-to-side rotation of the flexed lower extremities. This motion relaxes muscles that connect the lower extremities to the pelvis and relaxes muscles that connect the pelvis with the lumbar and thoracic spine. These motions should be performed slowly and initially through small ranges of motion. A key to successful use of these exercises is to limit the range of motion so that the patient does not feel stretching, but rather feels a relaxation into the available range of motion. If the therapist performs the activity, reductions in muscle tension will present as decreases in resistance to passive movement. Furthermore, as muscle tension decreases, the therapist will observe that

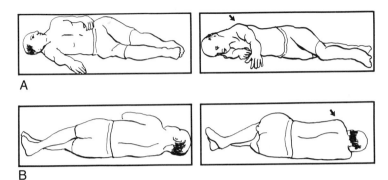

Fig. 9-11. In side-lying the thorax is slowly rotated forward and backward relative to the pelvis while the upper extremity is protracted and retracted relative to the thorax.

increasing numbers of vertebral segments participate in producing the rotational motion. With practice, the patient should be able to identify and reproduce decreases in tension.

In side-lying, rotation of the thorax on the pelvic complex and of the pelvic complex on the thorax are both important. The therapist should observe and guide these motions to ensure that as many intervertebral segments are relaxed as possible. The therapist's hand can be placed over the patient's iliac crest to prevent pelvic motion and to allow the patient to feel the dissociation of the thorax from the pelvis. Once the patient can reproduce the exercise, tactile cues from the therapist are unnecessary. Similarly, slow, rhythmic protraction and retraction of the scapula on the thorax can be used to relax the scapular musculature. These protraction/retraction exercises may be done most easily at first with the shoulder flexed and the elbow extended, so that relaxation of the total shoulder complex is addressed (Fig. 9-11). The therapist may need to guide the scapular movement with one hand while preventing the thorax from moving backward and forward with the other hand. Finally, the shoulder complex and thorax can be relaxed in combination by rhythmically moving the scapula and thorax forward and backward while the patient is side-lying.

Returning to the supine position, the entire cervical and shoulder-complex area can be relaxed as a unit. For this exercise, the shoulders are abducted to about 90° and the elbows flexed to 90°, and the arms and neck are then rotated rhythmically and slowly; the head is turned slowly from side to side in rhythm with the shoulders, which are internally and externally rotated. (Both shoulders may be symmetrically rotated internally and externally; alternatively, one shoulder can be internally rotated while the opposite shoulder is externally rotated) (Fig. 9-10B). This particular exercise serves to relax coordinately the entire chest area. If done properly, the patient and therapist should feel relaxation of the pectoralis muscles, internal and external rotator muscles of the shoulder, and latissimus dorsi, as well as of the cervical muscles, such as the sternocleidomastoid and the upper trapezius muscles. As the chest area relaxes, the therapist can guide the patient to "tuck the chin" and thereby reduce the forward head position.

Breathing exercises can be combined with the foregoing relaxation techniques in order to enhance the muscle relaxation and to increase the patient's vital capacity.[7] The breathing exercises should be initiated with the relaxation exercises after the patient has demonstrated a good ability to coordinate the breathing and rotational relaxation exercises separately. The key to all of the above exercises is to perform them slowly, within small ranges of movement, and to ensure that the patient is not using effort to move but rather is relaxing into the motion.

I have found that the above exercises are effective and efficient in relaxing the musculature of the neck and trunk to allow substantial rotational movement throughout the vertebral column. The efficacy of other relaxation techniques could also be investigated. It is possible that the same effects might be achieved with imaging, relaxation techniques, or the biofeedback techniques designed to reduce blood pressure and heart rate.[86] A recent case report supports the use of meditation to decrease dystonia.[87] The theoretical basis for attempting to achieve muscle relaxation through these techniques is the suggestion throughout the literature that muscle tone of the rigid type is influenced through the alerting mechanisms, and the supposition that relaxation reduces the level of alertness. There is no clear-cut evidence for or against this theory, although it is well known that anxiety heightens rigidity and general relaxation reduces rigidity.[55]

Range of motion in the trunk and neck should be restored at every intervertebral segment to the extent possible. Hence, it is important to use range-of-motion techniques that are very specific, as opposed to gross stretching techniques. Passive and active range-of-motion exercises in the supported position fit well with the relaxation techniques described above. The relaxation exercises described above can themselves be used to increase range of motion following the philosophy of Feldenkrais[88] that mobility is achieved through relaxation. When using relaxation in this way, it is important to increase the rotational range of motion gradually and only to the point of tightness, and never to the point of resistance at which stretching would be needed to continue the rotation. In this chapter the term *segmental strategies* is used to refer to active exercises in which the emphasis is on motion at each intervertebral segment. Thus, a patient might practice trunk rotation exercises in which much of the trunk moves as a unit and rotation occurs at only a few spinal segments. Alternatively, if the patient practices trunk rotation exercises using segmental strategies, then total trunk rotation would be limited to that range of total motion in which all of the spinal segments are able to participate. Although total motion may therefore be more limited initially, the motion achieved in the long term may be greater.

A related approach is to use gentle, passive positional stretching techniques. For example, a patient in the side-lying position can place a pillow under the mid-trunk areas to increase the lateral flexion of the thoracolumbar region. This position can be used effectively, for example, while the patient is watching television. An alternative approach to gaining increased range of motion of the trunk musculature is to use active or passive stretching techniques in which the patient or therapist attempts to stretch soft tissues through the application of force. Soft-tissue stretching techniques can be combined with joint mobilization techniques in the event that loss of joint mobility also exists. Traditional stretching techniques may be particularly useful for regaining full range of motion at the hip, knee, ankle, and elbow. In general, these techniques are likely to have the greatest long-term benefit if the patient rather than the therapist learns to perform them, so that they can be incorporated into a long-term exercise program. It is important to remember that PD patients are generally in their sixties, seventies, or even eighties. They therefore fall into an age group in which loss of mobility may have come from other conditions. Techniques should be modified appropriately in the light of any such pre-existing conditions.

There is at present no indication of whether relaxation or stretching is more effective for restoring range of motion in PD, although it is likely that elements of the relaxation approach combined with elements of the stretching and mobilization approach would be efficacious. What does seem clear, from kinesiology and mechanics, is that mobility should be achieved throughout the trunk, pelvic complex, shoulder complex, and neck. It also seems apparent that PD patients can be most specific and therefore effective in increasing their trunk and neck mobility when they perform their exercises in supported positions (e.g., supine, side-lying). In these supported positions the patient can focus on relaxation and range of motion of the trunk without simultaneously trying to control body position against the forces of gravity.

As the patient becomes proficient in performing the exercises described above, it is possible to incorporate more complex movement sequences into the physical therapy program in an attempt to address motor planning/programming dysfunction. The patient might, for example, perform an upper-extremity movement routine in coordination with a lower extremity routine. One exemple is to have the patient lie in the supine position with his or her lower extremities flexed, shoulders abducted to 90°, and elbows flexed. In this position the patient rhythmically externally and internally rotates the shoulders while coordinately letting the hips fall from one side to the other. This exercise may be made increasingly complex by coordinately incorporated side-to-side head rotation and breathing exercises, and by making the upper-extremity motions asymmetric so that one shoulder rotates internally while the opposite shoulder rotates externally (Fig. 9-10B and C). By systematically increasing the difficulty in coordination of the exercise, the therapist can challenge the patient's capacity for performing complex, integrated motor tasks. In side-lying positions such as that illustrated in Figure 9-11, the patient can rotate the head to look over the shoulder, can incorporate upper-extremity abduction with trunk rotation to bring the thorax toward the supine position, and can incorporate lower-extremity abduction, bringing the lower body toward the supine position, thus gradually initiating a complex rolling activity from the side-lying position.

There are several issues to consider in the sequencing of motor actions described above. First, the progression to this complex task should be developed gradually, so that the patient retains a capability for relaxed movement as the difficulty of the task increases. Second, the therapist and patient should pay close attention to the segmental motions involved in the task, insuring that the patient uses his or her full capacity for segmental mobility of the spine. Third, the task should be performed in a supported position so that the patient's attention can be directed at coordination of the motor aspects of the task without the added complexity of having to keep the body upright against gravity. With these concepts in mind, the variety of complex coordinated motor sequences available to the patient and therapist are limited only by imagination and the patient's capability for improving the sequencing of complex motor activities.

All of the exercises described above should lead to functional improvement. Hence, these exercises must be directly linked to functional tasks. The most obvious and essential functional activities in the positions described relate to mobility in bed and to rising from the supine to the sitting position. An essential step in this part of the exercise program is to practice rolling and rising to the sitting position with relaxed segmental motions that incorporate mobility throughout the spine. The patient strives to retain segmental rotational strategies while rolling. When coming to the sitting position, the patient incorporates lateral flexion in coordination with rotation of the spine. Ideally the patient should use these strategies automatically and without conscious control of their sequencing. If, however, the patient cannot relearn these mechanically favorable strategies automatically, then it is important to teach the patient to use conscious control and to deliberately choose segmental strategies of movement that incorporate rotation and lateral flexion of the spine. This will help to make the patient's function mechanically favorable for as long as possible, and to preserve intervertebral segmental mobility.

Specific Treatment Techniques in Sitting

Range of motion and coordination of the lumbopelvic area are essential for good balance control. The sitting position is excellent for addressing mobility and coordinated motion of this important area of the spine. Control of the lumbopelvic area should include anterior and posterior pelvic tilts achieved through extension and flattening of the lumbar spine, as well as lateral tilting of the pelvis to both sides through lateral flexion of the lumbar spine (Figs. 9-10 and 9-12). These motions can be facilitated through gentle anterior/posterior (Fig. 9-12A) and side-to-side (Fig. 9-12B) rocking motions with emphasis on lumbar mobility. As with the supine exercises, these motions should be done through very small ranges, with the range increasing as relaxation and mobility are achieved. Initially the therapist can cue and guide the patient with gentle hand pressure over the lumbar spine for anterior tilt and over the iliac crest for lateral tilt of the pelvis. Is it essential that the patient learn to differentiate rocking motions accomplished through lumbopelvic mobility from rocking motion accompanied by moving the trunk as a block. Motion of the pelvis accomplished through movement of the entire trunk is not segmental and is to be avoided. Rather, the patient's shoulders should remain in the midline position,

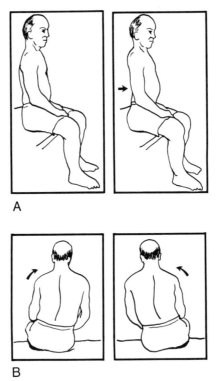

Fig. 9-12. Pelvic exercises in sitting. **(A)** The pelvis is anteriorly and posteriorly tilted while the shoulders remain midline. **(B)** The pelvis is laterally tilted (by lumbar lateral flexion) while the shoulders remain midline.

and pelvic motion should be accomplished primarily through lumbar spinal motion.

As the lumbopelvic area becomes more relaxed, the patient and therapist can begin active exercises to increase the range and coordination of pelvic motion. Initially the exercises should focus on increasing the control of anterior-posterior and side-to-side pelvic motions. As the range and control of these motions increase, the therapist should guide the patient in coordinated anterior, posterior, and lateral pelvic motions. The pelvis can be gently rotated clockwise, counterclockwise, or in figures-of-eight. (Feldenkrais[88] has designated this type of exercise the "pelvic clock exercises.")

These exercises can be modified by having the patient sit with the feet supported on the floor, elbows on a table in front, and head resting in the palms of the hands. In this position the spine can move only in a closed kinetic chain, so that rotational motions at the pelvis are translated upward throughout the spine. This position is excellent for relaxation of the entire trunk and neck area, in coordination with relaxation of the lumbopelvic area.

As the patient gains capability for the coordinated control of lumbopelvic mobility, the emphasis of the exercises can be modified to focus on automatic lumbopelvic adjustments for self-initiated and externally induced balance activities. For self-initiated activities, the patient or the therapist shifts the patient's weight from side to side, with the patient's attention focused on overall body displacement rather than specifically on the lumbopelvic motion. The therapist can meanwhile use appropriate handling techniques (such as tactile ones over the iliac crest and lumbar spine) to assure that automatic lumbopelvic mobility is facilitated. Finally, weight-shifting activities can be made more automatic and functional by having the patient practice tasks (e.g., reaching for items to the side or in front, bending over to tie shoes, rising from sitting to standing, etc.) while the therapist facilitates the appropriate postural adjustment through his or her hand placements.

In each of the foregoing activities, the patient focuses attention on the task at hand, so that the exercise is a goal-directed exercise. The therapist can use light tactile cues to the patient's lumbar spine and pelvis to facilitate automatic incorporation of the appropriate lumbopelvic motions that had previously been practiced as component motions under the patient's conscious control. If these component motions do not occur automatically during function, even with practice, it is important for the therapist to teach the patient strategies for using attention and conscious control whenever possible during function, to ensure safety and optimum functional independence.

Exercises for the sitting patient that can be adapted to the strategies outlined in this section have been described by a variety of authors.[19,88] The key to using any exercise in conjunction to this approach is to follow a few simple guidelines:

1. The patient should focus on relaxation rather than effort for movement.
2. The therapist should observe where motion is occurring within the patient's spine.
3. If motion does not occur throughout the spine, the therapist should decide whether the limitations responsible for this are fixed and beyond change, or whether exercises should be redirected to specifically gain relaxation and mobility of the immobile spinal segments.
4. An attempt should be made to facilitate the automatic incorporation of postural adjustments into all functional movements. If these adjustments do not occur automatically with repeated practice, the therapist and patient should decide whether the patient can use conscious control to ensure the use of segmental strategies of movement for functional activities such as reaching while sitting or rising from the sitting to the standing position. Only when it becomes impossible or unrealistic for the patient to use segmental strategies of movement should such compensatory techniques as rocking to initiate rising from the sitting to the standing position be encouraged.

Specific Treatment Techniques in Standing

The purpose of treatment techniques in the standing position is to facilitate coordinated movement with automatic balance control for walking and performing functional tasks. The treatment techniques used for this are similar to those described for more supported positions, beginning with relaxation, progressing to active movement, and culminating with the integration of automatic postural responses during functional movement.

Relaxation techniques can be used with the patient's feet parallel to one another or with one foot in front of the other. The arms may hang loosely at the patient's sides or may rest on a surface such as a desk or countertop. Slow rotational motions, analogous to those described for the patient in the sitting position, are performed. These techniques can be specifically focused to improve the mobility of the feet, lumbopelvic area, or trunk, depending on the instructions the therapist gives the patient and on whether the techniques are used in a closed kinematic chain by having the upper extremities supported and hence the trunk fixed at both ends.

Balance activities in the standing position may include responses to self-initiated displacements (e.g., reaching to the side, reaching with trunk rotation) or responses to externally induced perturbations (e.g., displacements from a rocking board or displacements applied by the therapist). The patient may also practice unilateral stance. Walking backward can be a useful technique for improving balance control in coordination with conscious motor acts. An ice-skating or waltzing movement can be valuable in assisting the patient to regain more coordinated integration of lumbopelvofemoral movement in stance for smoother patterns of movement.

Gait activities should include both walking for distance and the slow stepping that is used during many standing household tasks, such as dressing and cooking. In the case of walking for distance, an individual normally moves with a speed that requires a condition of continuous dynamic stability. Characteristics of this type of gait have been described for healthy individuals and can be used as a standard or basis of normal performance. The gait used in many household tasks is slower, with the emphasis on weight shifts from one inherently stable position to another. Practice of the 360° turn can be one useful preparation for this type of gait activity. Pre-gait type activities[19] can also be useful, particularly if they are incorporated into a functionally relevant sequence.

Miscellaneous Treatment Techniques

A few of the direct effects of PD are not specifically addressed by the interventional techniques outlined above. These include slowness in initiating and executing fine motor activities, difficulties with motor planning/programming for fine motor control, and tremor. There is sparse evidence for the effectiveness of physical therapy techniques in remediating the impairments that result specifically from pathology of the central nervous system. If physical treatment can improve these aspects of fine-motor dysfunction, it would seem that the same type of techniques used to measure reaction time, performance time, and motor planning/programming would be most appropriate. For example, the practice of tasks for hand function that require simultaneous execution of different motor programs might help to preserve a patient's capability in this area.

Tremor in PD has been particularly resistant to nonpharmacologic intervention, although there is one report suggesting improvement of tremor through physical intervention.[42] Palmer et al. demonstrated a reduction in tremor of as much as 42 percent with 14 PD patients in one of two exercise programs. One program consisted of exercises developed by the United Parkinson Foundation; the second consisted of upper-body karate exercises. It is unclear why or how tremor would improve through such exercises. It is important to note that Palmer et al.[42] measured tremor during a mental activation task as opposed to a functional activity. Furthermore, they did not report the initial extent of the tremor. Thus, the change reported is difficult to interpret. The observation of Palmer et al.[42] certainly deserves further study, to establish its reproducibility, determine whether tremor also improves during function, and determine why the exercises employed would reduce tremor.

Compensatory techniques should also be explored by the therapist and patient to improve fine-motor capability when tremor cannot be reduced through pharmacologic or physical intervention. The use of computers in place of handwriting as well as other assistive devices should be considered. Rosen and collaborators have taken an alternative approach to the management of upper-extremity tremor in PD.[89] They have begun development of an external damping device for the upper extremity. The device is designed to damp intention tremor and hence to improve the patient's capability for fine-motor function. Such an approach might ultimately prove of great benefit to PD patients for whom tremor is severely disabling.

Drooling and difficulty with voice projection are among the most socially disabling aspects of PD. Both impairments may be exacerbated by poor head/neck/thoracic posture and lack of mobility of the related muscles. Relaxation, muscle-lengthening, and coordination techniques should be modified to address the neck and facial areas.

Home and Group Exercises

Parkinson's disease is a chronic progressive disorder. It is neither feasible nor appropriate to provide PD patients with permanent physical therapy in a clinic setting. The long-term success of any physical therapy intervention for the ambulatory PD patient depends on the ability and commitment of the patient and/or the patient's family to continue the appropriate exercises at home. One of the most important aspects of physical therapy in PD is therefore patient education about appropriate posture, range of motion, appropriate movement, and the critical importance of continuing with necessary exercises.

The home exercise program should be specifically tailored to the individual needs of the patient. The interpretation of the patient's impairments and disabilities serves to guide the components of the formal physical therapy protocol. Appropriate exercises can be chosen from those used within the clinic setting.

Many of the exercises described in this chapter can be adapted for home use. A variety of less specific protocols are also available for general exercise for PD patients.[90,91] Exercises outlined in these pamphlets can be incorporated into the patient's home exercise program as appropriate for the particular individual.

Group exercise programs also can have a valuable place in the ongoing, early management of PD. Group exercise programs have the benefit of providing social and emotional as well as physical support to the patient.[92,93] They can be structured to provide support to both the patient and the family, which is an important aspect of the ongoing adjustment to PD.

EFFICACY OF PHYSICAL THERAPY INTERVENTION

The days of physical therapy intervention for PD without proof of efficacy are fast approaching. Furthermore, the importance of early physcial therapy intervention for prevention and correction of the impairments of PD is neither widely understood nor well established.[94-96] Indeed, some authors have specifically noted that physical therapy is not necessary early in the disease, and many authors suggest that the major role of physical therapy is for added support and to teach compensatory techniques for walking and transferring safely. It is imperative that the efficacy of intervention early in PD be established through careful and focused clinical observation, documentation, and experimentation.

A few investigators have reported on specific intervention programs for PD patients.[7,42,93,97] Palmer et al.[42] compared the benefit of two different 12-week exercise programs (an upper-body karate training program and a United Parkinson Foundation program). These investigators reported that both exercise programs resulted in improvements in gait, tremor, grip strength, and fine-motor control. They found no change in rigidity and reported a loss of function for whole-body coordination. Their study is an excellent example of the use of quantifiable, objective measures to determine performance before and after intervention. The results of the study illustrate that very different exercises can improve the function and ease the impairments of PD patients.

Stefaniwsky and co-investigators[97] studied the effects of different external sensory stimuli (visual, auditory, and touch) on improving the initiation time for an elbow-extension task in PD patients. They found an objective improvement of movement initiation time with all of these stimuli. They also reported subjective improvements in speech and gait, suggesting that at least some of the patients' gains could have been an effect of the attention given them rather than of the specific interventional methods chosen. These investigators did not report on upper-extremity function in relation to the sensory stimuli program.

Mitchell et al.[93] studied the effects of groups exercises on the performance of seven PD patients. They found improvements in mobility (measured with the mobility subscale of the Columbian Parkinson Scale) and perceived function (measured with a five-point Likkert-like scale).

These studies, directed at measuring the efficacy of physical therapy intervention in PD, should provide a challenge to other researchers and clinicians to document and critically explore the efficacy of physical therapy for the disease.

Several comments are in order about efficacy studies: first, PD is not a homogeneous disease. The impairments and disabilities of PD patients therefore may vary greatly. This has two ramifications for efficacy studies. The first is that treatment techniques should be designed to address specific impairments. Their efficacy should be tested with a group of patients in whom those impairments occur with similar severity. For example, Schenkman et al.[7] have provided a rationale for an intervention to ease the musculoskeletal impairments that occur indirectly from PD. These investigators provide two case studies illustrating the use of this exercise program for patients whose main impairments are musculoskeletal as a consequence of rigidity and bradykinesia. They have not yet reported experimental results in testing their approach.

Second, appropriate measurement is critical in efficacy studies. The evaluation techniques reviewed in this chapter are appropriate for measurement of many of the impairments caused by PD. Yet there are some impairments for which no good, objective clinical evaluation exists. For the most part, however, the evaluation process can be objective, as illustrated by the work of Palmer et al.[42] It is equally important that the exercise program be clearly and specifically described. This ensures that exercises tested experimentally can be used clinically. Finally it is important to measure the functional benefit of different exercises. If reaction time or motor programming is improved by various exercises in an experimental context, but there is no functional carryover, the value of the exercises must be questioned.

In summary, PD is a complex, multifaceted disease. It is time to address the specific impairments it produces with carefully focused intervention techniques. With further appropriate experimentation it will be possible to determine which impairments can be corrected through physical therapy, which can be prevented, and which require compensatory techniques. The model outlined in this chapter is intended to assist in focusing clinical physical therapy methods and experimental research in PD to permit these determinations.

REFERENCES

1. Webster DA: Critical analysis of the disability in Parkinson's disease. Med Treat 5:257, 1968
2. Hoehn MM, Yahr MD: Parkinsonism; onset, progression, and mortality. Neurology 17:427, 1967
3. Ilson J, Bressman S, Fahn S: Current concepts in Parkinson's disease. Hosp Med 19:33, 1983
4. Vincken WG, Gauthier MD, Dollfuss RE et al: Involvement of upper-airway muscles in extrapyramidal disorders. A cause of airflow limitation. N Engl J Med 311:438, 1984
5. Marsden CD: The mysterious motor function of the basal ganglia. The Robert Wartenberg Lecture. Neurology 32:514, 1982

 6. Mortimer JA, Pirozzolo FJ, Hansch EL, Webster DD: Relationship of motor symptoms to intellectual deficits in Parkinson's disease. Neurology 32:133, 1982
 7. Schenkman M, Donovan J, Wolfenden J et al: Management of individuals with Parkinson's disease. Rationale and case studies. Phys Ther 69:944, 1989
 8. Martinez-Martin P, Bermego-Parega F: Rating scales in Parkinson's disease. p 235. In Jankovic J, Tolosa E (eds): Parkinson's Disease and Movement Disorders. Urban and Schwarzenberg, Baltimore, 1988
 9. Feldman RG, Lannon MC: Parkinson's disease and related disturbances. p. 147. In Feldman RG (ed): Neurology: The Physician's Guide. Thieme Medical Publishers, New York, 1984
10. Diamond, Markham CN: Evaluating the evaluations: or how to rate a scale of Parkinsonian disability. Neurology 33:1098, 1983
11. Schenkman M, Butler RB: A model for multisystem evaluation, interpretation, and treatment of individuals with neurologic dysfunction. Phys Ther 69:538, 1989
12. Schenkman M, Butler RB: A model for multisystem evaluation and treatment of individuals with Parkinson's disease. Phys Ther 69:932, 1989
13. Massion J: Postural changes accompanying voluntary movements. Normal and pathological aspects. Hum Neurobiol 2:261, 1984
14. Critchley J MacD: Discussion on volitional movement. Proc R Soc Med 47:593, 1954.
15. Stein GM, Lander CM, Lees AJ: Akinetic freezing and trick movements in Parkinson's disease. J Neurol Trans (suppl) 16:137, 1980
16. Schenkman M: Interrelationship of neurological and mechanical factors in balance control. p. 29. In Duncan PW (ed): Balance. Proceedings of the APTA Forum. American Physical Therapy Association, Alexandria, Virginia, 1990
17. Steindler A: Kinesiology of the Human Body under Normal and Pathological Conditions. Charles C Thomas, Springfield, Illinois, 1955
18. Riegger C, Powers W, Foster J: Gross Anatomy Laboratory Manual. Weston Textbook Series, Northeastern University Custom Book Program, Boston, 1981
19. Bobath B: Adult Hemilplegia: Evaluation and Treatment. 2nd Ed. William Heinemann Medical Books, London, 1978
20. Gordon J: Assumptions underlying physical therapy intervention: Theoretical and historical perspectives. p. 1. In Carr JH, Shepherd RB (eds): Movement Science: Foundations for Physical Therapy in Rehabilitation. Aspen Publications, Rockville, Maryland, 1987
21. Schenkman M, Rugo de Cartaya V: Kinesiology of the shoulder complex. Journal of Orthopaedics and Sports Physical Therapy 8:428, 1986
22. Wood PHN: The language of disablement: A glossary relating to disease and its consequences. Int Rehab Med 2:86, 1980
23. Jette A: Functional disability and rehabilitation of the aged. Top Ger Rehab 1:1, 1986
24. Reynolds GP, Riederer P: The neuropharmacology of Parkinson's disease. p. 127. In Stein G (ed): Parkinson's Disease. Johns Hopkins University Press, Baltimore, 1990
25. Agid Y, Ruberg M, Raisman R et al: The biochemistry of Parkinson's disease. p. 99. In Stein G (ed): Parkinson's Disease. Johns Hopkins University Press, Baltimore, 1990
26. Burton K, Calne DB: Pharmacology of Parkinson's disease. Neurol Clin 2:461, 1984
27. Hallett M: Physiology and pathopysiology of voluntary movement. p. 351. In Tyler HR, Dawson DM (eds): Current Neurology. Houghton Mifflin, Boston, 1979

28. Jette AM, Davies AR, Cleary PD et al: The functional status questionnaire: reliability and validity when used in primary care. J Gen Intern Med 1:143, 1986
29. Murray MP, Sepic SB, Gardner BM et al: Walking patterns of men with Parkinsonism. Am J Phys Med 57:278, 1978
30. Murray MP, Drought AB, Kory RC: Walking patterns of normal men. J Bone Joint Surg 46A:335, 1964
31. Murray MP, Kory RC, Clarkson BH, Sepic SB: A comparison of free and fast speed walking patterns of normal men. Am J Phys Med 45:8, 1966
32. Inman VT, Ralson HJ, Todd F: Human Walking. Williams and Wilkins, Baltimore, 1981
33. Observational Gait Analysis Handbook: Ranchos Los Amigos. The Professional Staff Association, Downey, California, 1989
34. Van Sant AF: Rising from a supine position to erect stance. Descriptions of adult movement and a developmental hypothesis. Phys Ther 68:185, 1988
35. Nuzik S, Lamb RL, VanSant AF, Hirt S: Sit to stand movement pattern: A kinematic study. Phys Ther 66:1708, 1986
36. Schenkman M, Berger R, Riley PO et al: Total body dynamics in rising from sitting to standing. Phys Ther 70:638, 1990
37. Riley PO, Schenkman M, Mann RW, Hodge WA: Mechanics of a constrained chair rise. J Biomech 24:77, 1991
38. Tinetti ME: Performance-oriented assessment of mobility problems in elderly patients. J Am Geriatr Soc 34:119, 1986
39. Holden MK, Gill KM, Magliozzi M et al: Clinical gait assessment in neurologically impaired. Reliability and meaningfulness. Phys Ther 64:35, 1984; J Am Geriatr Soc 34:119, 1986
40. Patla AE, Winter DA, Frank JS et al: Identification of age-related changes in the balance control system. p. 43. In Duncan PW (ed): Balance. Proceedings of the APTA Forum. American Physical Therapy Association, Alexandria, Virginia, 1990
41. Wing AM, Keele S, Margolin DI: Motor disorder and the timing of repetitive movements. Ann NY Acad Sci
42. Palmer SS, Mortimer JA, Webster DD et al: Exercise therapy for Parkinson's disease. Arch Phys Med Rehab 67:741, 1986
43. Nakamura R, Taniguchi R: Dependence of reaction times on movement patterns in patients with Parkinson's disease and those with cerebellar degeneration. Tohoku J Exp Med 132:153, 1980
44. Bloxham CA, Mindel TA, Frith CD: Initiation and execution of predictable and unpredictable movements in Parkinson's disease. Brain 107:371, 1984
45. Flowers K: Ballistic and corrective movements in an aiming task. Intention tremor and Parkinsonian movement disorders compared. Neurology 25:413, 1975
46. Day BL, Dick JPR, Marsden CD: Patients with Parkinson's disease can employ a predictive strategy. J Neurol Neurosurg Psychiatry 47:1299, 1984
47. Kendall FP, McCreary EK: Muscles. Testing and Function. 3rd Ed. Williams & Wilkins, Baltimore, 1983
48. Braun BL, Amundson LR: Quantitative Assessment of head and shoulder posture. Arch Phys Med Rehab 20:322, 1989
49. Koller WC, Glatt S, Vetere-Overfield B, Hassanein R: Falls and Parkinson's disease. Clinical Neuropharmacology 12:98, 1989
50. Coughlin L, Templeton J: Hip fractures in patients with Parkinson's disease. Clin Orthop Rel Res 148:192, 1980
51. Staeheli JW, Frassica FJ, Sim FH: Prosthetic replacement of the femoral head for

fracture of the femoral neck in patients who have Parkinson's disease. J Bone Joint Surg 70-A:565, 1988

52. Traub MM, Rothwell JC, Marsden CD: Anticipatory postural reflexes in Parkinson's disease and other akinetic-rigid syndromes and in cerebellar ataxia. Brain 103:393, 1980

53. Viallet F, Massion J, Massarino R, Khalil R: Performance of a bimanual load-lifting task by Parkinson's patients. J Neurol Neurosurg Psychiatry 50:1274, 1987

54. Dietz V, Berger W, Hostmann GA: Posture in Parkinson's disease. Impairment of reflexes and programming. Ann Neurol 24:660, 1988

55. Rogers MW: Motor control problems in Parkinson's disease. p. 195. In Lister MJ (ed): II Step: Contemporary Management of Motor Control Problems. Proceedings of the II Step Conference. Foundation for Physical Therapy, Alexandria, Virginia, 1991

56. Dick JPR, Rothwell JC, Berardelli A et al: Associated postural adjustments in Parkinson's disease. J Neurol Neurosurg Psychiatry 49:1378, 1986

57. Horak FB, Nashner LM, Nutt JG; Postural instability in Parkinson's disease: Motor coordination and sensory organization. Soc Neurosurg Abstr 10:634, 1984

58. Teravainen H, Calne DB: Studies of Parkinsonian movement: Initiation of fast voluntary eye movement during postural disturbance. Acta Neurol Scand 62:149, 1980

59. Tinetti ME, Williams TF, Mayewski R: Fall risk index of elderly patients based on number of chronic disabilities. Am J Med 80:429, 1986

60. Ashburn A: Physical therapy assessment for stroke patients. Physiotherapy 68:109, 1982

61. Carr JH, Shepherd RB, Nordhold L et al: Investigation of a new motor stroke assessment scale for stroke patients. Phys Ther 65:175, 1985

62. Horak FB: Clinical measurement of postural control in adults. Phys Ther 67:1881, 1987

63. Wusteney E: Center of Gravity Control as a Measure of Balance. Master's Thesis. MGH Institute of Health Professions, Boston, 1990

64. Dettmann MA, Linder MT, Sepic SB: Relationships among walking performance, postural stability, and functional assessments of the hemiplegic patient. Am J Phys Med 66:77, 1987

65. Gordon VC, Oster C: Rehabilitation of the patient with Parkinson's disease. JAOA 71:307, 1974

66. Rothwell JC: Control of Voluntary Movement. p. 310. Aspen Publishers, Rockville, Maryland, 1987

67. Dietz V, Quintern J, Berger W: Electrophysiologic studies of gait in spasticity and rigidity. Evidence that altered mechanical properties of muscle contributes to hypertonia. Brain 104:431, 1981

68. Jankovic J: Pathophysiology and clinical assessment of motor symptoms in Parkinson's disease. p. 99. In Koller WC (ed): Handbook of Parkinson's Disease. New York, Marcel Dekker, 1987

69. Watts RL, Wiegner AW, Young RR: Elastic properties of muscles measured at the elbow in man: II. Paients with Parkinsonian rigidity. J Neurol Neurosurg Psychiatry 49:1177, 1986

70. Talland GA, Schwab RS: Performance with multiple sets in Parkinson's disease. Neuropsychologia 2:45, 1964

71. Brown RA, Lawson DA, Leslie GL, et al: Does the Wartenberg pendulum test differentiate between spasticity and rigidity? A study in elderly stroke and Parkinson's patients. J Neurol Neurosurg Psychiatry 51:1178, 1988

72. Watts RL, Wiegner AW, Young RW: Elastic properties of muscles measured at the elbow in man: II Patients with Parkinsonian rigidity. J Neurol Neurosurg Psychiatry 49:1177, 1986
73. Knuttson E, and Mårtensson A: Quantitative effects of L-Dopa on different types of limb movements and muscle tone in Parkinson's disease. Scand J Rehab Med 3:121, 1971
74. Meyer CH: Akinesia in Parkinsonism. Relation between spontaneous movement (other than tremor) and voluntary movements made on command. J Neurol Neurosurg Psychiatry 20:582, 19
75. Fahn S, Tolosa E, Marin C: Clinical rating scale for tremor. p. 225. In Jankovic J, Tolosa E: Parkinson's Disease and Movement Disorders. Urban and Schwarzenberg, Baltimore, 1988
76. Hallett M, Kloshbin S: A physiologic mechanism of bradykinesia. Brain 103:301, 1980.
77. Brooks VB: The Neural Basis of Motor Control. Oxford University Press, New York, 1986
78. Sharpe MH, Cermak SA, Sax DS: Motor planning in Parkinson patients. Neuropsych 21:455, 1983
79. Daniels L, Worthingham C: Muscle Testing. Philadelphia, W B Saunders, 1972
80. Norkin C, White DJ: Measurement of Joint Motion: A Guide to Goniometry. Philadelphia, FA Davis, 1985
81. Youdas JW, Carey JR, Garrett TR: Reliability of measures of cervical spine range of motion. A comparison of three techniques. Phys Ther 71:98, 1991
82. Dillard J, Trafimow J, Andersson GBI et al: Motion of the lumbar spine. Reliability of two measurement techniques. Spine 16:321, 1991
83. Estenne M, Hubert M, Troyer A de: Respiratory muscles movement in Parkinson's disease. N Engl J Med 311:1516, 1984
84. Bogaard JM, Hovestadt A, Meerwald J et al: Maximal expiratory and inspiratory flow-volume curves in Parkinson's disease. Am Rev Resp Dis 139:610, 1989
85. Gentile AM: Skill acquisition: Action, movement and neuromotor processes. p. 93. In Carr JH, Shepard RB (eds): Movement Science for Physical Therapy in Rehabilitation. Aspen Publishers, Rockville, Maryland, 1989
86. Benson H: The Relaxation Response. Avon Books, New York, 1975
87. Szekely BL, Turner SM, Jacob RG: Behavorial control of L-DOPA induced dyskinesia in parkinsonism. Biofeedback Self Regul 7:443, 1982
88. Feldenkrais M: Awareness through Movement: Health Exercises for Personal Growth. Harper & Row, New York, 1972
89. Bergenhause S, Rosen MJ, Huang S: Evaluation of a damped joystick for people disabled by intention tremor. p. 41. RESNA 12th Annual Conference, New Orleans, LA, 1989 (abstract)
90. United Parkinson Foundation: Exercise Program. Chicago, United Parkinson Foundation, 1984
91. LaVigne J, Roberts KM: Home Exercises for Patients with Parkinson's Disease. American Parkinson Disease Association, New York, 1982
92. Szelekey B, Kosanovich NN, Sheppard W: Adjunctive treatment in Parkinson's disease. Physical therapy and comprehensive group therapy. Rehab Lit 43:72, 1982
93. Mitchell PH, Metz MA, Catanzaro ML: Group exercise: A nursing therapy in Parkinson's disease. Rehab Nursing 12:242, 1987
94. Greer M: How to achieve maximum benefit for the patient with Parkinson's disease. Geriatrics 31:89, 1976

95. Perlik SI, Koller WC, Weiner WJ et al: Parkinsonism: Is your treatment appropriate? Geriatrics 35:65, 1980.
96. Weiner WJ, Singer C: Parkinson's disease and nonpharmacologic treatment programs. Am Ger Soc 37:359, 1989
97. Stefaniwsky L, Bilowit DS: Parkinsonism: Facilitation of motion by sensory stimulation. Arch Phys Med Rehab 54:75, 1973

10 | Final Comments

George I. Turnbull

In 1987, at the World Confederation of Physical Therapy Congress in Sydney, Australia, the idea that a book should be written about the physical therapy treatment of Parkinson's disease (PD) was hatched by Margaret Sharpe and myself. We agreed that PD was a neglected condition in the physical therapy world but that the need was significant. In addition, we both agreed that a meaningful role for the physical therapist existed but that some of the assumptions governing the practice of physical therapy would have to be laid aside. The primary purpose of this book has been to raise questions but also to propose some possible answers.

It is interesting to contrast what has been written about physical therapy in PD compared with stroke. Volumes exist proposing novel and innovative ways to treat the disabilities caused by cerebrovascular disease. The work of Brunnstrom, Bobath, Lane, Carr and Shepherd, Cotton and Kinsmen and Johnston are but a few examples of the intense efforts to find more satisfactory treatment approaches to a condition that disables so many people. Patients suffering from PD have not been so lucky in terms of physical therapy endeavor to seek solutions to this common and equally disabling disorder. Perhaps this has resulted from the euphoria created by the highly successful management of the disease by medication. Many physicians are under the impression that the pharmacologic approach has obviated the need for physical therapy, and physical therapists have tended to accept this conclusion, probably because PD patients are not easy to deal with nor are rewarding because they do not get better. It is time, however, in the light of new knowledge, to scrutinize this practice, analyze current methods and propose new approaches to this problem. This has been an objective of this book.

The target audience of this book, according to the editorial board, are physical therapists who have been practicing for 10 years or so. As a result, a number of different perspectives, which is symbolic of the multidisciplinary approach to this disease, have been presented. In addition, attempts have been made to allow the physical therapist to try and identify, on a personal level,

193

with the difficult-to-understand symptoms of PD. Studying the disease from a medical and physiologic perspective is a common practice and is important, but personalizing the symptoms as human beings is likely to lead to considerable insights into the functional impact of this disorder and what it means for our patients to live like this on a daily basis. Only with this sort of empathy will the motivation be generated to attempt to seek practical solutions on a meaningful level.

The suggestion that physical therapists consider a different role from the one to which they normally subscribe has been a recurrent theme in various parts of this book. The role of the physical therapist as a provider of care, an assessor, a resource, and an educator are all highly achievable objectives. This is particularly true if the therapist accepts the premise that it may not be necessary to be with the patient to create an impact. This is an age of technologic explosion. Camcorders are affordable. Patients have videocassette recorders linked to their televisions at home. Computers have enormous potential for helping PD patients. This is particularly true of those computers capable of high-quality desk-top publishing techniques and programs that can store and access custom-made information. The booklet in Chapter 8 was produced by these techniques. It provides the patient with a guide so that exercises can be done in the comfort of the home at a frequency that will result in motor learning. The aim of this approach is to preserve functional competencies for as long as possible.

For this approach to be successful, the provision to the patient of clearly written and illustrated home exercise routines is an absolute necessity. Physical therapists have had experience with home exercise prescription for a very long time. Usually, the exercises are written down and pretyped for the patient. The therapist goes to a bank of materials and selects the exercises that are most appropriate for the patient. This works well until the material runs out or the exercises are not quite right for the patient.

To get around these types of problems, this author is developing the concept of being able to access a bank of exercises and resource materials that can be tailor-made for each patient but in a manner that is not time intensive. The procedure involves the use of HyperCard, a system of organizing information that uses the Apple MacIntosh computer. By writing a number of stacks that are readily accessible using on-screen buttons, information can be stored and retrieved very readily (Fig. 10-1). For example, a stack of exercises or information would be prepared ahead of time and stored in the computer in a number of stacks. The stacks relevant for a particular patient, following careful assessment, can then be called up, modified when necessary, and printed out in a visually pleasing manner. Using this technique, it is possible to supply only relevant information to the patient rather than redundant material that provides details of symptoms from which the patient does not suffer, a practice that can lead to confusion and the receipt of false impressions. Further, the provision of written materials that are not directly applicable to the patient is not efficient educational practice. In addition to these features, the resource material can be personalized with the patient's name in the same way as commercial companies

Mrs Churchill Livingstone

HELPful

Exercises for

Living with

Parkinson's disease

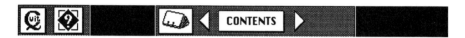

CONTENTS

Fig. 10-1. HyperCard cover page, which can be customized to include patient's name.

personalize advertisements—an effective method of gaining attention. Again, this enhances patient motivation and compliance.

Figure 10-1 shows the cover page as presented in HyperCard. Notice that this card has been customized for Mrs. Churchill Livingstone. Clicking on the Contents button reveals the information, or Table of Contents, in the HyperCard stack (Fig. 10-2). A further click on any one of the words in the Table of Contents reveals the card clicked. As an example, clicking on Helpful Hints will call up the card shown in Fig. 10-3. The content of that card is the same as that contained in the booklet described in Chapter 8.

Thus, a customized information bank can be constructed, the relevant portions of which can be printed out for each individual patient. Similarly, any alteration of the generic information contained on the cards can be carried out quickly and with an ease that shatters the myths surrounding the complexity of the computer. It is proposed that when the education of the patient is a priority and descriptions of exercises must be conveyed in a manner that will ensure their accurate replication during home exercise routines so that motor learning will occur, this medium is easy to use and possesses significant potential.

Sway Platform

Another innovation being developed at this time to enhance the provision of home exercise routines is a sway platform. Although originally designed to enhance balance in stroke patients, this device has the potential to be used

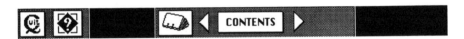

Table of Contents

PD Facts
Introduction
Benefits of an Exercise Program
Role of Physiotherapy
Posture
Breathing
Exercises
Balance/Walking
Relaxation Techniques
Helpful Hints
Work Sheet Record

> Click on the
> section that you
> wish to see

Fig. 10-2. HyperCard Table of Contents. Clicking on any item will immediately call up that section of the material.

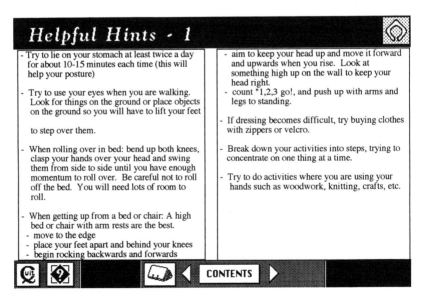

Helpful Hints - 1

- Try to lie on your stomach at least twice a day for about 10-15 minutes each time (this will help your posture)

- Try to use your eyes when you are walking. Look for things on the ground or place objects on the ground so you will have to lift your feet to step over them.

- When rolling over in bed: bend up both knees, clasp your hands over your head and swing them from side to side until you have enough momentum to roll over. Be careful not to roll off the bed. You will need lots of room to roll.

- When getting up from a bed or chair: A high bed or chair with arm rests are the best.
  - move to the edge
  - place your feet apart and behind your knees
  - begin rocking backwards and forwards

- aim to keep your head up and move it forward and upwards when you rise. Look at something high up on the wall to keep your head right.
- count "1,2,3 go!, and push up with arms and legs to standing.

- If dressing becomes difficult, try buying clothes with zippers or velcro.

- Break down your activities into steps, trying to concentrate on one thing at a time.

- Try to do activities where you are using your hands such as woodwork, knitting, crafts, etc.

Fig. 10-3. The card that appears when Helpful Hints is clicked.

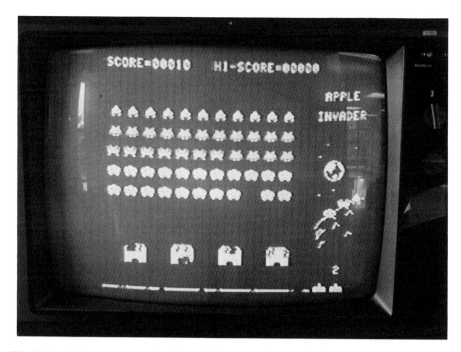

Fig. 10-4. The screen seen by the patient while playing a commercially available video game. The patient manipulates the spaceship by shifting his centre of pressure and fires a gun, which is operated by hand to kill the aliens.

with PD patients to improve the speed and accuracy of balance responses, particularly when the subject is still ambulant. The objective in PD would be to encourage the patient to rehearse regularly postural responses, thus preserving their efficiency. A low-cost microcomputer-based sway platform system, which determines the instantaneous centre of pressure beneath the feet, has been built and is currently being tested. The platform interacts with a simple computer, through the game port, and can be used instead of a joystick to control video games (Fig. 10-4). This system has also been developed to measure certain aspects of balance performance that permit quantification of change over time. Although similar systems are currently available, their considerable cost limits use to only the most affluent of physical therapy departments and certainly eliminates them as a home exercise option. This system is specifically designed to be inexpensive and thus can be considered to be viable both for use in physical therapy departments and as a home exerciser. The device has both treatment and assessment capabilities.

Treatment Function

A patient who is using this device as a treatment would place both feet on the platform, either in a standing or a sitting position. The patient then

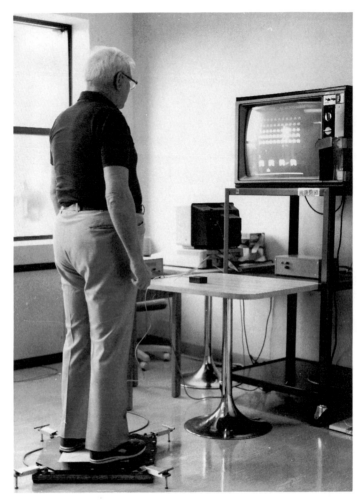

Fig. 10-5. A subject rehearsing postural responses while fighting for survival against evil aliens. (From Turnbull GI, Wall JC: Gait reduction following stroke: the application of motor skills acquisition theory. Physiotherapy Practice 5:123, 1989, with permission.)

plays a commercially available videogame, undertaking postural responses in the direction of the desired movement by manipulating the position of the cursor on the video screen (Fig. 10-5). Thus, movement in both the sagittal and frontal planes is encouraged with the success or failure of their efforts during the game and by the total score obtained. This would encourage the rehearsal of postural responses while the feedback ensures that motor learning is enhanced.

Exercises are thus made more enjoyable and challenging and can be individualized to meet the particular needs of a given patient. This factor may help to overcome the problem of compliance, which confounds many minimally supervised exercise programs, particularly when the exercises are of extremely repetitive and subject to boredom, as they tend to be in long-term programs. Although not yet incorporated, it is also possible to have the computer monitor the frequency of home exercises patient performance, thereby providing the attending physical therapist with an accurate record with which to assess progress as well as compliance. In addition, improvements in performance would be associated with a higher score achieved on the computer game.

Measurement Function

The sway platform interfaced with an Apple IIe microcomputer can also be used to determine the location of the centre of pressure of subjects in standing position and to determine the ability of subjects to manipulate the center of pressure. The mean position of the center of pressure is calculated in both the X and Y axes along with the standard deviation from the mean for each during any part of the data collection period. The mean value provides information concerning the position of the center of pressure of the subject while the length of the line traced by the center of pressure over the data collection period provides the magnitude of postural sway. The standard deviation provides an indication of the magnitude of the variance from the mean. These data can provide information concerning postural steadiness of the subject.

Although this device is in the early part of its development, it provides a useful example of the type of innovation necessary to deal with patients with long-term disabilities needing long-term home exercise routines. To achieve the repetition of exercises with the accurate feedback necessary to permit motor learning to occur and without the presence of the physical therapist, it seems that this type of approach might be successful. Although balance responses are the motor behaviors targeted in the system just described, similar technology exists by which all sorts of additional movement combinations could be rehearsed and thus, in the PD patient, preserved for as long as possible.

Two examples have been provided to illustrate methods to cope with the ongoing physical therapy management of the patient with PD. There is a need to vigorously pursue further innovations so that the person suffering from this disease can be better served by the physical therapy community in a manner afforded the person disabled by stroke. To achieve this objective, creativity, problem-solving capabilities, and a strong measure of imagination need to be combined with the more traditional neurophysiologic, neuroanatomic, and motor control theories to begin to build a comprehensive and effective approach to the management of the person with PD. There is little question that there will be further advances in the pharmacologic management of this condition, and it will be interesting to see the results of the carefully controlled fetal neural tissue transplantation experiment currently being carried out at Dalhousie University. Nonetheless, these advances will not eliminate the need for physical therapy management of PD. On the contrary, maintaining the patient in top physical condition for as long as possible will likely become a top priority. Thus, the physical therapy community must respond. It is unlikely that the solutions to this problem will come from one source. As a result, we must all strive to reason solutions to problems and then communicate the results in the literature. Only then will the whole become greater than the sum of the parts.

In striving for this objective, we must not, however, lose the human face on our patients. I first met Moira MacPherson four years ago. A fellow Scot, who had developed PD some years ago, she remains an inspiration to others and myself. Her tragedy has been my tragedy, but she has never backed down. Her greatest joy is to be demonstrated to students and remain asymptomatic for the duration of the presentation. With her husband, Peter, she has been instrumental in building the Halifax PD community into a national force. It is my intention to finish this book with Moira's words, which are eloquent in describing something of which many of us are aware and yet, at the same time, know nothing.

The Dark Side of the Moon

On the dark side of the moon, breathing is difficult, communication almost impossible.

My body lies in awkward angles of rigid immobility. Only the tears of helplessness and frustration flow easily, and my hands drift upwards, following some unconscious need to touch my face. I am suddenly aware of them, and they freeze and hang claw-like and useless. My husband gently presses them back to my sides. "Another pillow?" I concentrate and manage a jerky irritable "No." I sense his anguish and hurt that there is nothing he can do to help me. I want to tell him to leave so that he need not feel my despair, but I have stopped communicating. I have become a totally selfish, self-centered being with all my dwindling energies needed to keep myself breathing and keep holding up the weight of my inwardly collapsing skeleton. This is the darkest shadow, the bottom of the "low."

In the distance I hear Peter telling me not to fight it, "Just relax and it will be over sooner." Why do I have to keep telling him that it's impossible to relax with a body that feels like a crudely constructed meccano . . . or does it? . . . I can feel the drugs start to work—a creepy crawling feeling of hundreds of worms just beneath the skin, then ecstasy as my neck muscles start to relax. I can feel my legs. Life is returning.

In a bedroom filled with sunlight, we laugh as I bounce up and down on the bed and wriggle and stretch and vow, once again, never to take normal movement for granted.

A friend of mine died yesterday. She spent much of her last weeks on the "dark side of the Moon," but as I write this, the first warm glow from the rising April sun spreads softly across my desk and I know she is free and smiling in the sunlight.

(Reprinted by kind permission of the author.)

Index

Note: Page numbers followed by f indicate figures, and those followed by t indicate tables.